Contents

Chapter ONE

INTRODUCTION

From the desk of Bill Campbell,

The prospect of losing our eyesight is one of the scariest things we can imagine. The ability to soak in the exquisite beauty of the world around us, with its myriad vibrant colors, is something we take for granted...

until it starts to slip away from us.

That's why I'm so glad that you have put your faith in me with your purchase of **The Outback Vision Protocol**.

You see, if your vision is failing, then you don't have a lot of time to follow false trails, try dead-end methods or chase pie-in-the-sky rainbows.

For you, **time is running out**.

So, if you've noticed that your eyesight keeps getting worse and you don't know why...

If you're concerned about whether the deterioration will ever stop, and would like to put the brakes on before you lose your eyesight completely and become a burden to your family...

If you ever get embarrassed or frustrated at your inability to read or see things properly...

If you like the idea of saving thousands of dollars on future eye care costs...

If you're experiencing blurry vision, blind spots, 'floaters', specks, or any kind of issue with your vision that simply shouldn't be there...

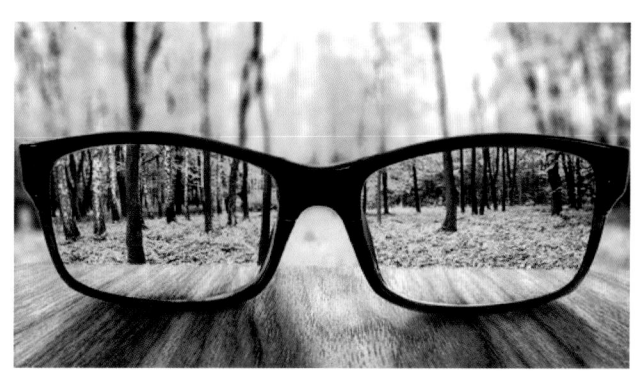

And if you want a scientifically proven way to correct your failing eyesight and achieve perfect 20/20 vision in as little as three weeks…

Then you have just made what may turn out to be the **wisest investment of your entire life**.

Within these pages, you are about to discover a clinically proven, all-natural protocol that will allow you to achieve crystal clear, *20/20 super sight* permanently.

And you will be able to do it without the aid of corrective lenses or dangerous surgery – or even those pointless eye exercises that are all over YouTube.

What's more, you'll be able to achieve these astounding results in **as little as 21 days**!

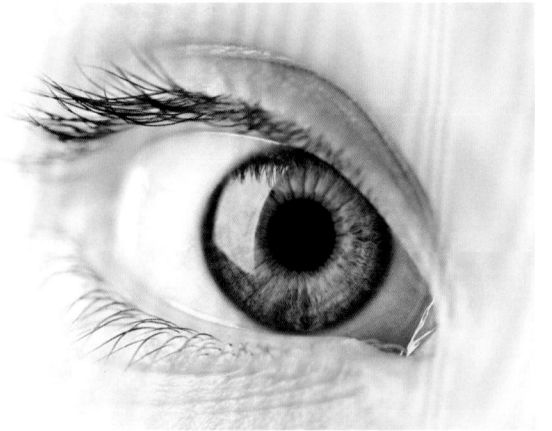

So, how are we going to do it?

Well, unlike the vast majority of so-called vision 'cures', we will forget about treating the symptoms of your vision loss and go directly to the root cause of the problem…

Free Radical Damage

You are about to discover how you can actually feed your eyes **eight crucial antioxidants** that will destroy those sight-robbing free radicals and restore your vision to crystal clear perfection in a matter of days.

OK, I know that right about now you're feeling skeptical.

How can such a remarkable turnaround take place in such a short period of time?

Well, let me tell you – if I hadn't seen the transformations, first with my lovely wife Lindsay, and then with literally thousands of volunteer test subjects, I'd be first in line in the skepticism queue.

But you simply cannot argue with results.

*So, all I ask is that you **put your skepticism aside for the next 21 days** and follow this course to the letter. If you are not astounded by the improvements in your vision, simply return this book for a no-questions-asked refund.*

You've got nothing to lose – but your eyesight!

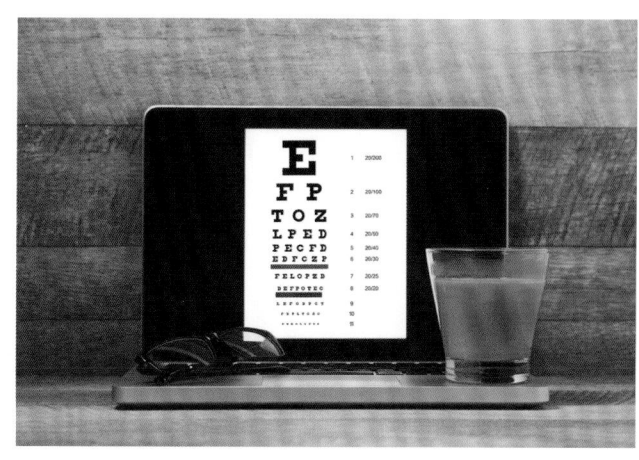

So, let's start getting yours back.

- Bill

CHAPTER TWO

HOW YOUR EYES WORK

Your vision is one of your most valuable tools, and certainly one you would miss if you lost it. Unfortunately, vision problems are extremely common. Though vision problems affect millions of people, many who have these problems don't fully realize it.

As your vision worsens over time, it is easy to get used to it – your body learns to adapt. However, if you let your vision continue to deteriorate, one day you may lose it completely and it may not be possible to get it back. So, if you want to preserve or restore your vision, you've come to the right place!

In this protocol, you'll learn everything you need to do over the next 21 days to restore your perfect vision. Before we get into the details, however, let's start with a simple quiz. Ask yourself the following questions to get a feel for the current state of your vision:

1. When looking at a television or computer screen for an extended period of time, do you find that your eyes become strained?

2. Do you find yourself blinking frequently or rubbing your eyes to clear your vision?

3. Can you clearly read text printed on billboards from 100 yards away?

4. Do you find yourself squinting when using your distance vision to identify things?

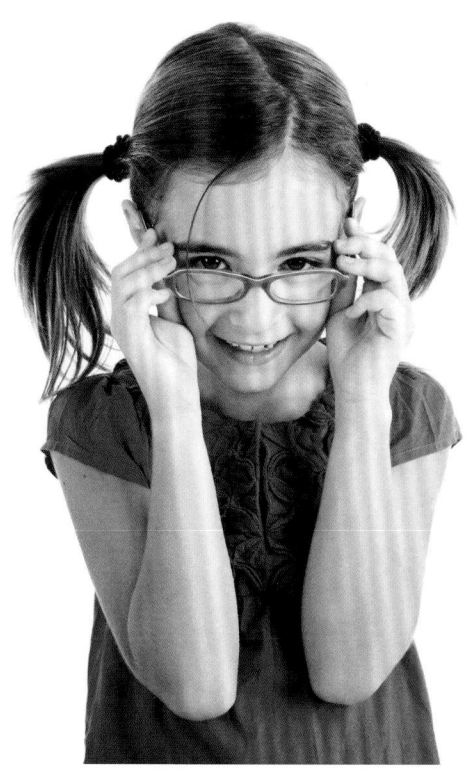

5.   Are you only able to read for short periods of time before your eyes become sore or your vision blurs?

6.   Do you experience motion sickness or nausea when driving or riding in a car?

7.   Are your eyes very sensitive to light or glare?

8.   Do you see rainbows or halos around bright lights, particularly at night?

9.   Is your vision sometimes limited by floating spots on the edges of your vision?

10. Do you sometimes experience double vision?

If you answered "Yes" to one or more of these questions, it could be a sign that you've experienced some changes to your vision. This test is not designed to diagnose any vision problems – it merely serves to increase your awareness of your own vision and how it may have changed over the years.

Now that you have a better idea of what kind of shape your eyes are in, let's start getting into the details for this vision-restoring protocol. The first step is to learn how your eyes work so you can understand how certain vision problems affect your eyes. From there, we'll move on to the real cause of your vision loss.

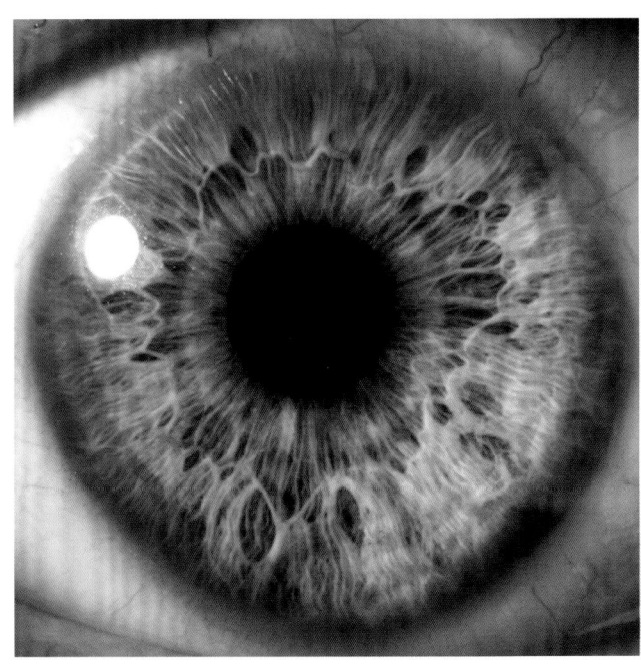

How Your Eyes Work

Each of your eyeballs is a beautiful machine with a lot of different parts that work seamlessly together to let you see. Poets say the eyes are the window to the soul, but the window to the eyeball is the cornea. This is a dome of clear tissue on the front of the eye. The cornea focuses light as it passes through.

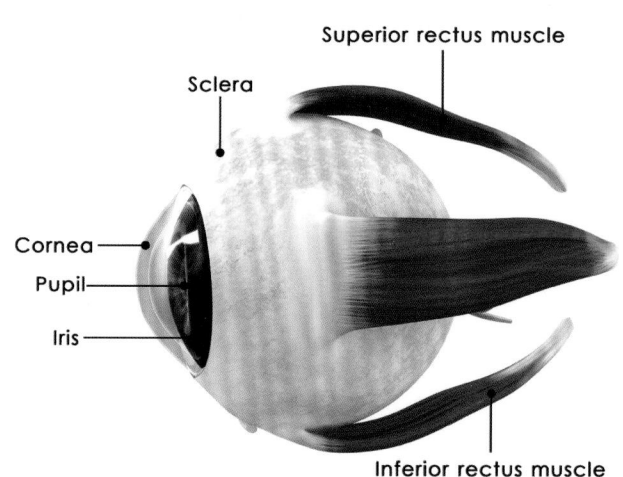

Superior rectus muscle
Sclera
Cornea
Pupil
Iris
Inferior rectus muscle

The lens is held in place by a bunch of fibers that attach to the ciliary muscle. This muscle changes the shape of the lens to allow for a change of focus, depending on whether the thing being looked at is close by or far away. To see something near, the ciliary muscles makes the lens thicker; to see something far away, it makes the lens thinner.

The colorful part of the eyeball is called the iris. It sits right behind the cornea. In the middle of the iris is a black circle called the pupil. This is an opening that lets light into the eye. The iris has muscles attached to it that can change in size. This makes the pupil bigger and smaller in order to control how much light gets through. The pupil gets smaller when there's a lot of light and bigger when it gets dimmer.

Once the light has passed through the cornea and the pupil, it passes through the lens. This is very similar to the lens in a camera. The lens focuses the light onto the back of the eye. Just like a camera lens, the lens in your eye is able to focus on things that are both close and distant.

From the lens, we travel to the retina, which is the back wall of the eyeball. The lens focuses the light onto the retina. The retina contains millions of light-sensitive cells called rods and cones. There are 129 million rods and 7 million cones in a healthy retina.

The rods see in black, white and shades of grey. They also help us to see the

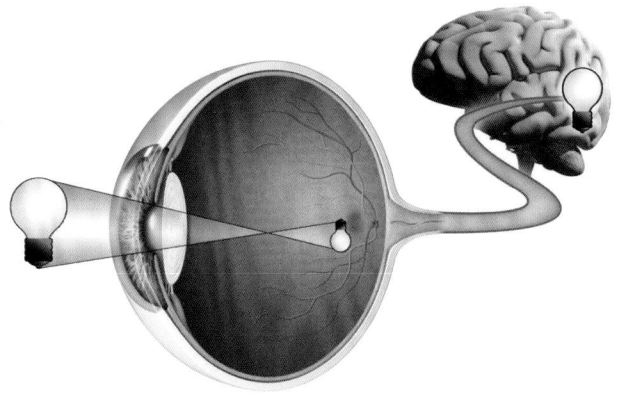

shape and form of a thing. Rods also help us to see in the dark. Cones, on the other hand, are sensitive to one of three colors – red, green or blue. Together, they let us see millions of colors. But cones need more light than rods to work with.

Behind the retina is the optic nerve. It carries messages to the brain about what you are seeing. Rods and cones convert the colors and shapes you see into millions of nerve messages. Those messages are then carried along the optic nerve to the brain. It's as if your eye is sending your brain a report on what you're seeing. The brain then 'translates' the report into whatever it is that you are looking at.

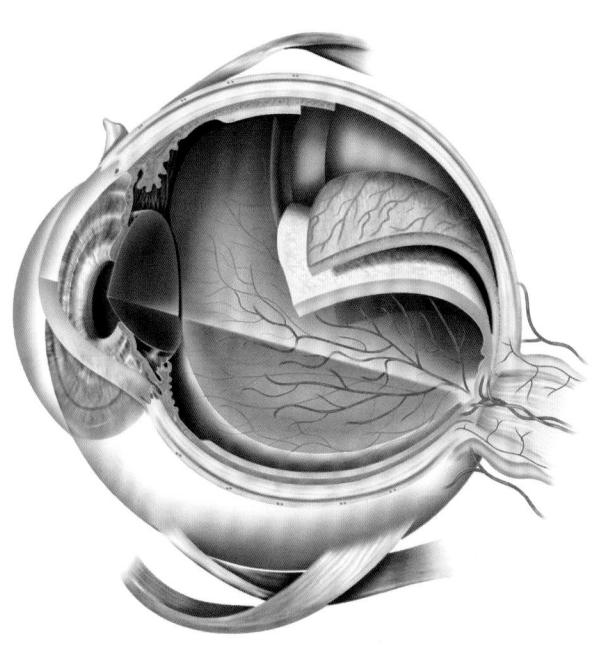

Focusing on Different Parts of the Eye

Sclera

The sclera is a tough outer coating of the eye that protects the entire eyeball.

Choroid

The choroid is a vascular layer of the eye. It contains blood vessels that nourish the inner parts of the eye.

Cornea

The front portion of the eye, the cornea, is convex in shape and bulges outward. Light enters the eye through the cornea.

Iris

The iris is a dark, muscular diaphragm located just behind the cornea. It regulates the amount of light entering the eye by adjusting the size of the pupil.

Pupil

The pupil is a hole in the middle of the iris. The pupil contracts or expands depending upon the intensity of light entering the eye.

Lens

The lens of the eye is made of a transparent jelly-like substance that is comprised of proteins. It is held in position by the ciliary muscles and suspensory ligaments, which are also known as ciliary zonules.

The ciliary muscles and suspensory ligaments adjust the focal length of the lens so that we can see both distant and nearby objects clearly. The ability of the eye to focus on distant and nearby objects by changing the focal length is called 'accommodation.'

Aqueous Humor

Aqueous humor is a gelatinous liquid in the area between the cornea and the eye lens. It prevents the eye from collapsing due to changes in atmospheric pressure.

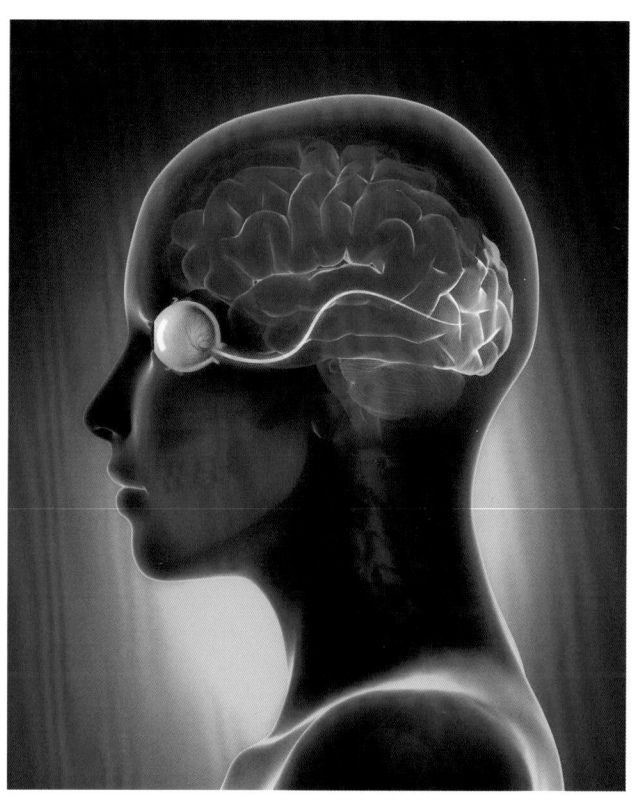

Retina

The retina is a delicate membrane that contains a large number of light-sensitive cells. These light-sensitive cells get activated upon illumination and generate electrical signals. There are two types:

- Rods, which are cells that respond to the intensity of light.
- Cones, which are cells that respond to the color of objects.

An inverted real image of the object is formed on the retina. The electrical signals generated by the cells are sent to the brain through the optic nerve.

Blind Spot

Your blind spot is a small region in the retina where the optic nerve enters the eye. It is called the blind spot because it is insensitive to light.

Macula

The macula is a tiny area in the retina that is responsible for clear and sharp vision. There is a small depression inside the macula called the 'fovea centralis.' Here, the maximum number of cones are present.

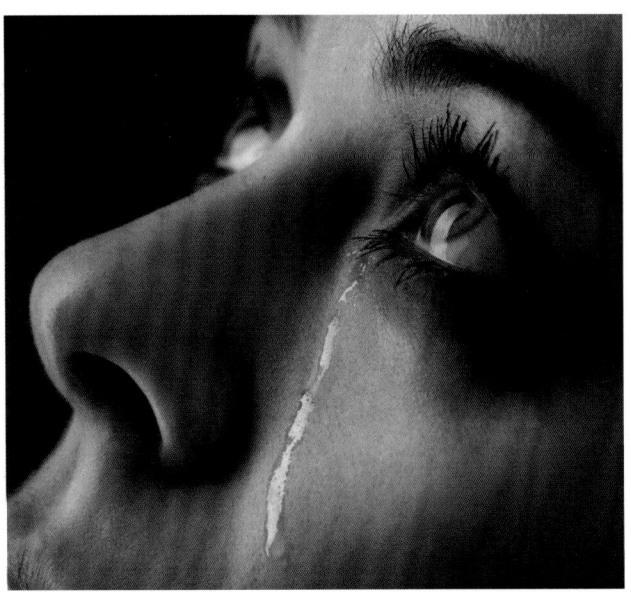

The Value of Tears

You actually have three different types of tears:

- Basal
- Reflex
- Emotional

Each type is brought on by different stimuli. However, they are all formed in the same way. Between your eyeball and eyelid sits the lacrimal gland. This gland produces and drains your tears. But before the tear is removed, you blink and spread it over the cornea. This coats your eye with liquid.

Basal tears have the job of keeping your cornea from drying out. They are always present and cover your eye in water, oil and mucous. On average, humans produce five to 10 ounces of basal tears per day.

Reflex tears are the type of tears that show up when an irritant gets in your eyes, such as smoke or onions. When this happens, the cornea sends signals to the brain telling it that you need more lubrication. As a result, you cry. These tears are mostly comprised of water. If there is too much for the eye-drainage system to handle, they spill out onto your cheeks.

The third group of tears are emotional. As your limbic system and hypothalamus process an intense emotion, they activate the autonomic nervous system, which you cannot control. This causes the heart rate to quicken, sweat to be released and tears to fall. Emotional tears contain the stress hormone ACTH as well as Enkephalin, a natural painkiller. This is why it sometimes feels relaxing to have a good cry.

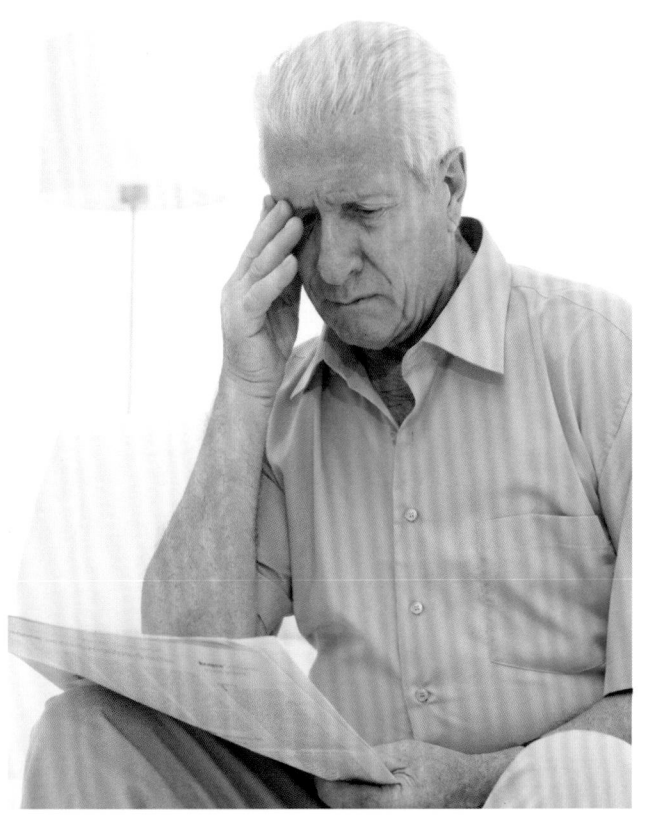

Researchers don't fully understand why crying has come to be a response to intense emotion. It is thought that crying can be a way to appear more vulnerable or submissive to an attacker. It is also a way to put your emotions on display, which elicits the help and support of friends and family.

Common Eye Problems

Now that we know how the eyes work, let's take a look at what happens when they don't. What follows are the most common eye problems and their causes. We'll also take an in-depth look at two of the most common causes of vision loss: glaucoma and macular degeneration.

Glaucoma

Glaucoma results from damage to the optic nerve, which is typically caused by abnormal pressure inside your eye. Glaucoma is among the leading causes of blindness in the United States.

Macular Degeneration

There are two types of macular degeneration:

- Dry
- Wet

Dry macular degeneration is the more common of the two. This eye disorder causes sight loss in the center of your field of vision.

Keratitis

Keratitis is a rare but serious eye problem that occurs when a type of amoeba invades the cornea. Often, these come from contaminated swimming water. Poor contact lens hygiene can also cause this eye infection that can threaten your eyesight.

Amblyopia (Lazy Eye)

Lazy Eye is a condition where one eye

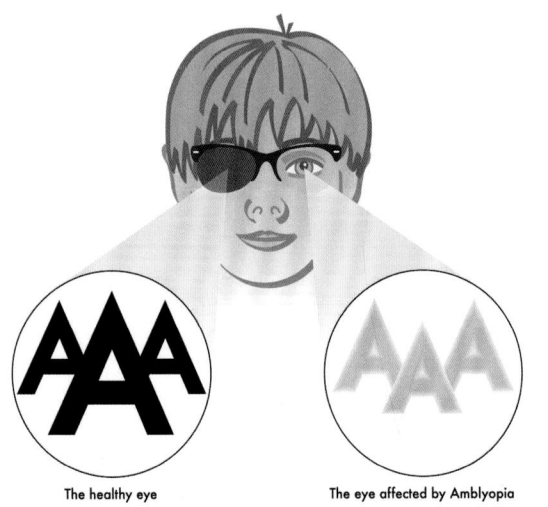

The healthy eye   The eye affected by Amblyopia

dominates the other. Amblyopia usually develops in young children. It can lead to permanent eyesight problems if not treated early.

Blepharitis

Blepharitis is an inflammation of the eyelids. It is one of those eye problems that sometimes results from a low-grade bacterial infection or skin disorder. It can cause chronic eye irritation, tearing and crusty debris. It can also make you feel as if you have a foreign body in your eye.

Cataracts

This occurs when proteins in the lens of your eye clump and causes cloudy vision. Cataracts happen mostly in the elderly, and can be corrected with surgery to replace the natural lens with an artificial one.

Color Blindness

This condition is characterized by an inability to tell color differences. Color blindness is usually inherited, but may also occur because of eye, nerve or brain damage; it may also occur as a result of exposure to certain chemicals.

Corneal Ulcer

Also known as ulcerative keratitis, a corneal ulcer is an open sore on the cornea. It is commonly called an eye sore. It may be caused by injury, dryness resulting from lack of tear production, or infection.

Detached Retina

Sometimes the retina, the light-sensitive membrane covering the back wall of the eyeball, peels away from its underlying layer of support tissue. A detached retina is a serious eye problem that requires immediate attention. Symptoms include flashes of light and floating spots.

Dry Eye

There are a number of conditions that can cause dry eye syndrome. Usually, this occurs when the tear-flow system of the eye is out of balance. However, it can also result from environmental factors.

Occlusions

Occlusions are sometimes referred to as eye strokes. A clot or blockage

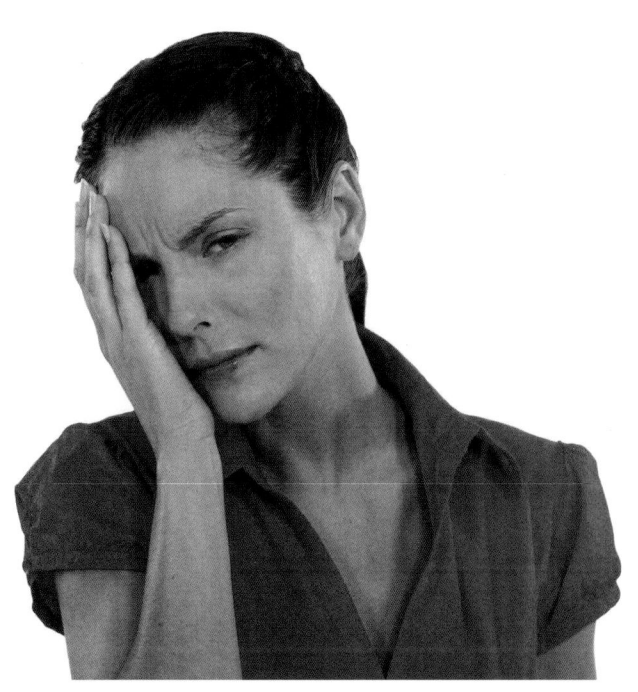

interrupts blood flow to parts of the eye, causing sudden vision damage.

Eye Twitching (Tic)

There are many possible causes of eye twitching. Twitching and tics may also be called 'eye spasms' or 'blinking disorder.'

Eye Floaters and Spots

Eye floaters are generally harmless, and occur in many people over the age of 40. They cause tiny blurry spots in your field of vision.

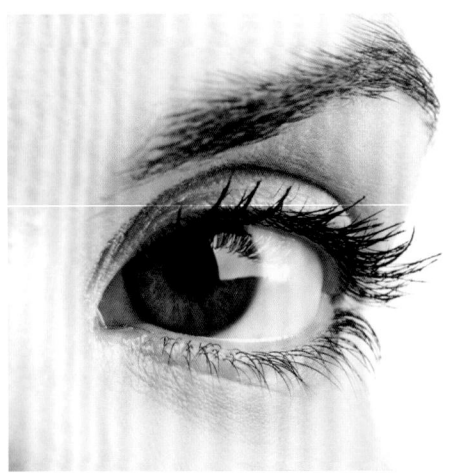

Macular Hole

This often happens in the elderly and people with disabilities. Vision suddenly becomes blurry or distorted.

Ocular Migraine

This is a common but incorrectly used term for an ophthalmic migraine. It is usually painless, but can be frightening because it gives you the sensation of looking through shattered glass.

Optic Neuritis and Optic Neuropathy

This is an inflammation of the optic nerve that can cause pain, blurry vision and blind spots. It may develop in an hour, or over the course of several hours.

Photophobia

This disorder is better known as light sensitivity. It is often caused by eye damage like a corneal abrasion, or when the pupil can't constrict normally and too much light is let in.

Strabismus

Strabismus is more commonly called 'crossed eyes.'

Eye Stye

An eye stye is an eye irritation that resembles a sore, pimple or boil that grows in the skin surrounding the eye.

Subconjunctival Hemorrhage

This eye problem results from a broken blood vessel of the white part of the eye. The eye suddenly becomes reddened.

Conjunctivitis

Conjunctivitis is an infection that is widely known as 'pink eye.'

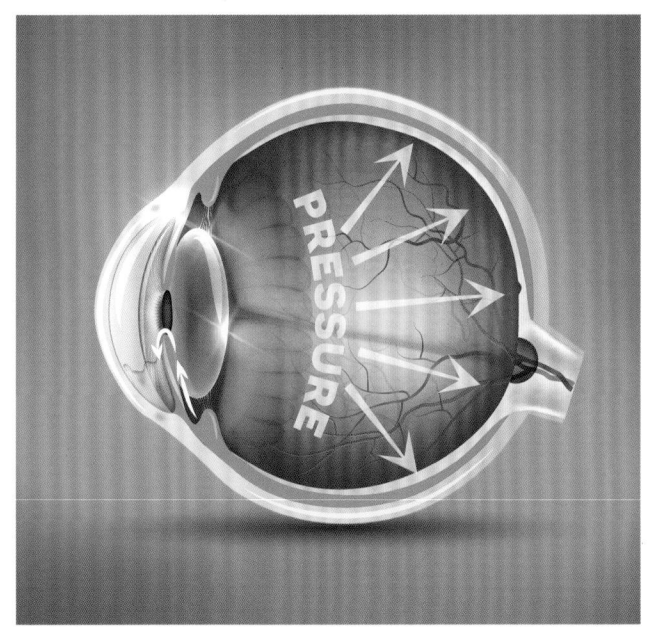

Focus on Glaucoma

The group of eye diseases collectively known as glaucoma is the most prevalent of all eye disorders. It affects about 66 million people around the globe each year. Of those, about 5 million become totally blind.

To understand what glaucoma is, we need to learn a little more about our eyes. The eye is able to maintain its rigidity through pressure. The soft tissues in the eye are pumped up, just as you would pump up a balloon. The 'pump' is the ciliary body and it causes aqueous humor to flow from the blood vessels into the eye. This aqueous humor is able to move around the eye,

providing it with nourishment. It then returns to the bloodstream by way of a strainer-like structure called the 'trabecular meshwork.'

It is when this meshwork becomes blocked that problems begin to occur. It causes the pressure inside the eye to go up. Over time, the delicate nerve fibers at the rear of the eye will suffer damage. This is what is referred to as 'open-angle glaucoma.' Ninety percent of glaucoma cases are of this type.

The pressure that is exerted inside the eye is constantly fluctuating. Such things as your heartbeat, how hydrated you are and the position in which you are sitting all affect this pressure. While high intraocular pressure is one sign of glaucoma, it should be noted that eye pressure can vary from person to person.

Angle-closure glaucoma is an acute, but rare, form of the condition. It is caused by a sudden increase in the amount of pressure in the eye. This is very painful and results in severe pain in the eye, dizziness and vomiting. It needs to be immediately treated to prevent blindness.

Secondary glaucoma is brought on by other eye conditions, such as eye injuries or cataracts. Congenital glaucoma also affects a small portion of the population. Present from birth, babies with the condition will have enlarged eyeballs.

Glaucoma is an insidious eye condition. It can creep up on us and overtake us without our even being aware of it. It does this with the aid of the blind spot, which we all have. This area is at the back of the retina, where the nerve fibers form to create the optic nerve. There are no light sensing cells at this point. The amazing brain, however, is able to fill in this blind spot, so we are not aware of the gap in our vision.

Glaucoma causes damage to the nerve structure surrounding the blind spot. It does this without giving out any signs of what is going on, such as dry or watery eyes.

There is currently no single, comprehensive test for glaucoma. Usually, an eye specialist will begin by checking the level of fluid pressure in the eye. He will also look for damaged tissue in the nerve structure between the brain and the eye.

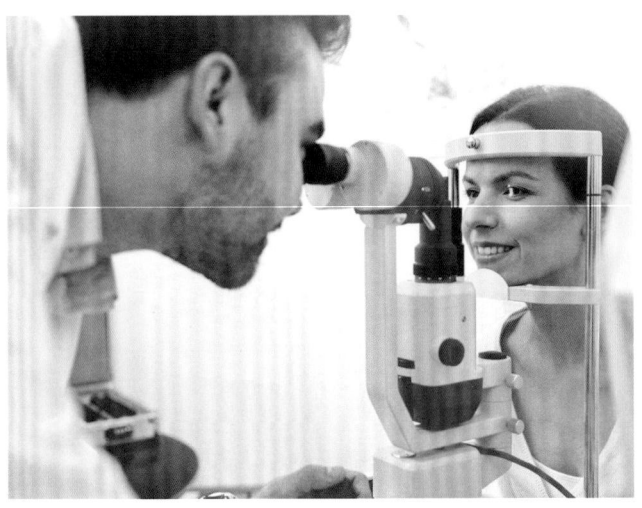

The strongest risk factors for glaucoma are the following:

- Being over the age of 45
- Being of African descent
- Having a family member who has the condition
- Having diabetes
- Being nearsighted
- Being a regular user of corticosteroids
- Having a previous eye injury

Conventional treatment for glaucoma involves using an eye drop a couple of times per day. These drops prevent the buildup of aqueous fluid in the eyeball. Laser treatment is another option. During this process, a laser beam is used to drill tiny holes in the front of the eye to allow for drainage. This helps to stabilize the pressure in the eye.

About Macular Degeneration

Another of the most common eye problems is age-related macular degeneration (AMD). This condition develops when the macula, part of your retina, becomes damaged, and it results in the loss of your central vision. When you develop macular degeneration, you lose the ability to see fine details, but your peripheral vision may remain unchanged. For example, if you were looking at a clock face, you might be able to see the numbers around the edges of the clock, but not the hands of the clock.

There are two types of macular degeneration: dry and wet. Dry AMD accounts for 80% of the people who have macular degeneration. It occurs when parts of the macula become thinner over time and small clumps of protein (called drusen) grow, obstructing your central vision.

Wet AMD is less common than dry AMD, but it is more serious. This form of macular degeneration occurs when new, abnormal blood vessels start to grow under your macula. These vessels start to leak fluid (such as blood), which causes scar tissue to develop on the macula. With wet AMD you also lose your central vision, but it happens more quickly.

Anyone can develop macular degeneration, but some of the risk factors may include the following:

- Caucasian (white) ethnicity
- Overweight or obesity
- Smoking cigarettes
- Family history of macular degeneration
- Over 50 years of age
- Eating a diet high in saturated fat
- Having heart disease or high cholesterol

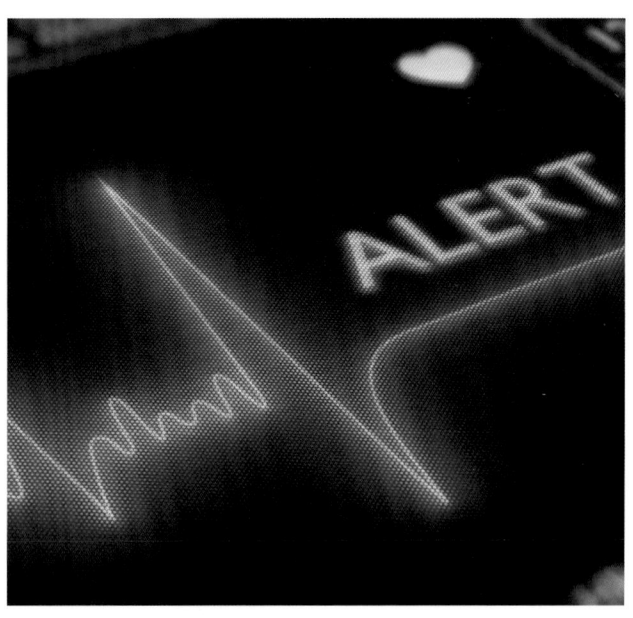

If you have one or more of these risk factors and you've experienced changes in your vision, it may be worth talking to your ophthalmologist. Macular degeneration is diagnosed through an eye exam involving an Amsler grid, as well as a regular eye exam to look at the internal structures of your eye. The Amsler grid helps to identify any spots or blurry areas in your field of vision.

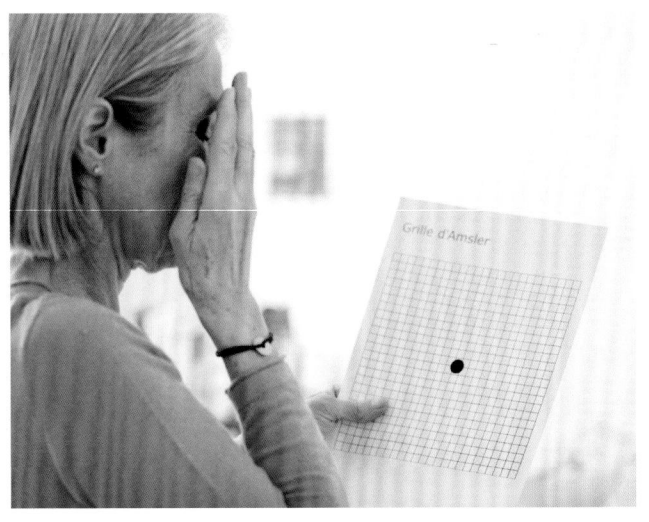

Treatment for macular degeneration is tricky – it is usually aimed at reducing symptoms because eliminating the underlying cause is not always possible. There are no effective treatments for dry AMD, but taking certain nutritional supplements, such as vitamins A and C, as well as lutein and zeaxanthin, may help to slow the progression. For wet AMD, treatment usually involves anti-VEGF drugs, which reduce the number of abnormal blood vessels under the retina and slow down any leaking fluid. Laser surgery is also a treatment option for some forms of wet macular degeneration.

CHAPTER **THREE**

FREE RADICALS – THE REAL CAUSE OF VISION LOSS

In this chapter, you are about to discover the real cause of vision impairment that has been robbing people of their precious sight without them even realizing it. While you have been relying on the conventional wisdom of the medical community, this silent stealer of sight has been pulling the wool over your eyes, leaving you shrouded in darkness.

Our journey to uncover this root cause begins with a couple of words that may cause your eyes to glaze over…

Free Radicals

You've probably heard these words before, but if you're like most people, you have no idea what they are or what they have to do with your eyesight. But before we find out that vital link, we need to take a step back and think about the importance of cellular nutrition.

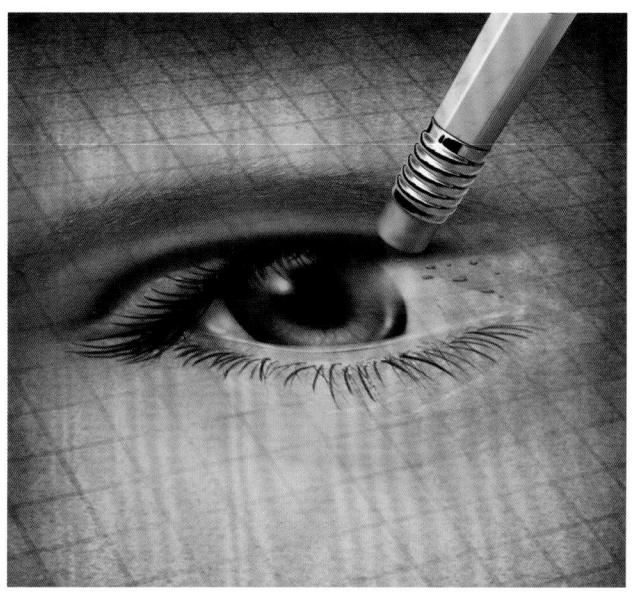

Toxic Cells

Cells are the building blocks of all living things. The word 'cell' derives from the Latin for 'small house.' Cells are the tiniest units that can replicate by themselves. Your body is composed of about 75 trillion cells, which make up all of the tissues that make you, you. For your cells to operate optimally, they need to be able to absorb the right nutrients from the right foods.

However, many of the cells in your body are not absorbing the nutrients that are being supplied to them. That's because they are clogged up with toxins (poisons), which are preventing the vitamins and nutrients from getting into them.

Toxins are all around you. In fact, you take them into your system with every breath you take. Processed foods contain all manner of toxins that contaminate and clog up the cells inside your body. So, day after day, year after year, toxins are building up in your body, preventing your cells from utilizing the nutrients that you are providing it. When we consider that most people are hardly doing a good job of taking in the essential vitamins and nutrients that their body requires, the fact that most of that pitiful amount isn't getting through is truly frightening.

The way to address this cellular deprivation is by focusing on what can be termed 'cellular nutrition.' Cellular nutrition focuses on working with your body's cells. It cleans them up, allowing them to become activated back to healthy operation. By addressing issues at the cellular level, we are able to overcome issues that may have been holding you back for decades. Your eyes will be able to more efficiently use the nutrients that are supplied to it, you'll have more energy and you will feel that you have reclaimed your deteriorating vision.

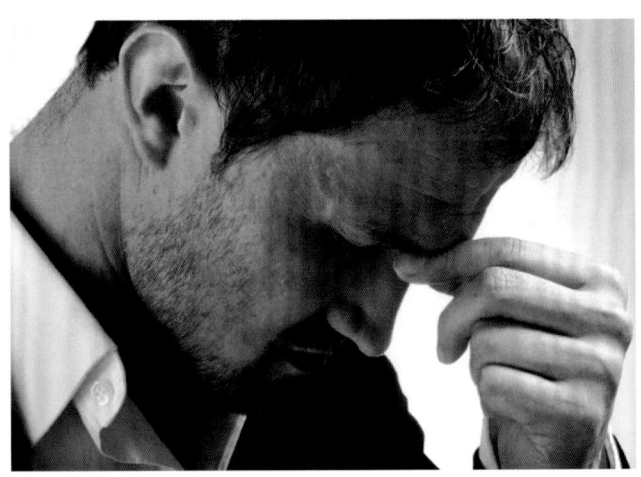

Oxidative Stress

Oxidative stress is a complicated process. Simply stated, it is what happens when the body's cells come into contact with oxygen. Oxygen has the effect of burning an electron from our molecules, making them unstable. An unstable molecule – which is what we call a 'free radical' – tends to act a bit crazy, bouncing around inside your cells and causing damage to them. Unless these unstable molecules are neutralized, the cells will degenerate.

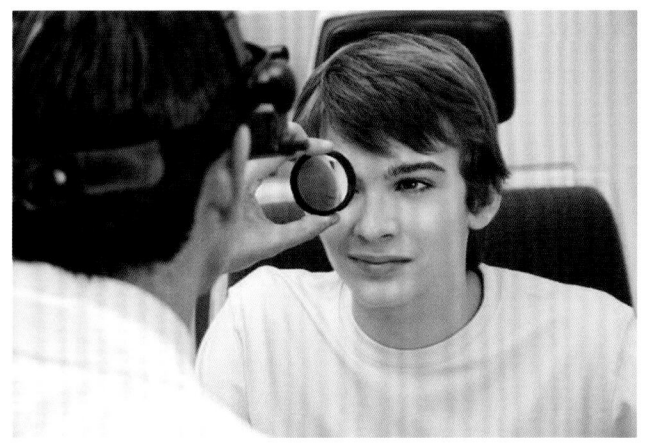

The result is that you will feel tired, lethargic and in pain.

So, what causes oxidative stress? The simple acts of breathing and eating will do it. When the air you breathe is pristine and the foods you eat are free of preservatives, the oxidative stress is minimized. Few people, however, enjoy pristine conditions or are able to consistently eat cleanly. For most people, then, oxidative stress is a problem. It leads to cell membrane damage and the accumulation of toxins. This, in turn, causes inflammation. Other factors also contribute to oxidative stress. Smoking, excessive alcohol consumption, taking prescription drugs, taking in pesticides, antibiotics and hormones through animal food sources and exposure to waterborne pollutants all play a part.

The Effects on the Eyes

The major visual problems, such as macular degeneration, glaucoma and cataracts, are caused by oxidative stress, which is, in turn, a result of free radical activity.

Free radicals destroy proteins, enzymes and DNA (1). This causes chronic damage to the tissues in and around the eyes. The eye is the most sensitive area of your body, which is why free radical activity in it can be so damaging. The retina is especially vulnerable to free radical damage (2).

This damage is the real reason that you are losing your vision.

Chapter **FOUR**

WHY GLASSES AND CONTACTS ARE NOT THE ANSWER

As a society, we take it for granted that wearing glasses is what we do when we have vision problems. Not many of us have given any serious consideration to what actually takes place when we put glasses on.

The eyes are constantly changing. Over the course of a day, they can become tired, with the result that we find it hard to focus.

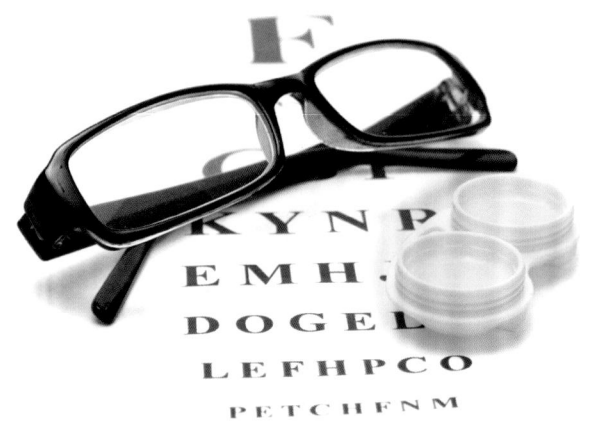

We wear glasses in order to fix refractive problems. The lens of the glass is designed to focus the thing that we are looking at on the retina at the back of the eye. The glasses compensate for the refractive error in the eye. However, unlike the eye itself, they do this in a constant, rather than a flexible, way. So, when we wear the glasses, the level of refractive error needs to be maintained in order for us to clearly see objects through the glasses.

For instance, if you get a pair of glasses with a 100% correction at the time of measurement, the problem becomes worse. It will force your eyes to constantly adapt to the conditions that were present at the time that your eyes were tested. In other words, if you went in for your eye test in the evening, every time you put on your glasses, your eyes are being forced to adapt to these conditions – even if it is early in the morning!

That is why many people complain that their eyes hurt when they first put on a new pair of glasses. The answer that they invariably get is that the pain will go away after a few days, when the glasses have been 'broken in.'

So, how does this affect your eyes?

The eyes are constantly being forced to adapt to the refractive error that was the case when your eyes were tested. That means that you are forcing your eyes to become worse in order for the glasses to work!

Many people use minus lenses for reading. Unfortunately, this actually makes your vision worse.

In order to be able to read at a normal reading level, nearsighted eyes must overaccommodate three diopters. A diopter is the power of the lens that is needed to correct your vision to normal (20/20 or metric 6/6); the higher

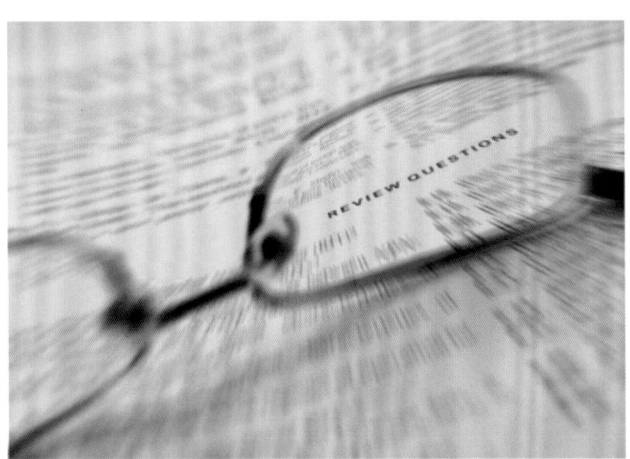

the number, the stronger the lens. However, a person who wears minus three diopter glasses in order to correct distance vision and keeps them on for reading, are putting their eyes under a huge amount of challenge – now they have to adjust for the three diopters needed by normal eyes to read AS WELL as the minus three diopters that are built into the lenses. So, they have to compensate for a whopping six diopters!

That's why you should never wear glasses that are created to improve long distance vision for reading. The additional strain on the eyes is damaging to your eyesight.

Nearsighted glasses are created to provide clear vision from 20 feet. The glasses are static, meaning that they don't adjust for conditions. So, if you use these glasses for reading something that is just a foot from your eyes, the words will be 20X out of alignment.

Technology can do a lot of wonderful things, but as of yet, it cannot produce a pair of glasses that is able to adjust its power as you go from reading a book to looking at a sunset.

That makes glasses a source of strain for your eyes.

All glasses are made with a lens that has just a single point of best vision. This is called the optic center of the lens. This point of best vision is located at the dead center of the lens – and the assumption is that you are always looking through this central area of the glasses.

But that is not the case. Your eyes are constantly moving, and you often look out through the off-center parts of the glasses. When you do this, the glasses act similarly to prisms. The effect of this is that the edges of the lenses get distorted. So, you are encouraged to keep your eyes locked in on the optic center of the glasses.

In order to help provide some flexibility in vision, some glasses are fitted with strong plus lenses. However, these end up being even worse for your long-term eyesight.

When you look out at the horizon, your eyes will look directly through the optic center of the glasses. Then, when you concentrate on the words of the page in front of you, you turn your eyes downward. This means that you will no longer be looking through the optic center of the glasses, which will place additional strain on the eyes.

Wearing nearsighted glasses while working on a computer will also be a problem for your eyes. The glasses will not be adjusted to allow you to read at a foot with a book and to work at two feet on the computer. This will place additional strain on your eyes.

Studies back up the contention that glasses can be detrimental to eyesight. One study, conducted at New York University, saw biologists fitting lenses on young primates and analyzing how their vision was affected. It was shown that wearing a minus lens actually caused elongation of the eyeball.

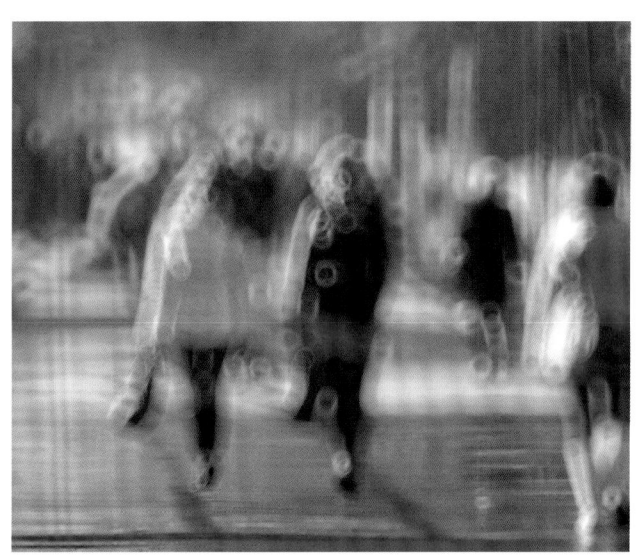

Nearsightedness is the result of an elongated eyeball, so wearing glasses actually caused nearsightedness to get worse (3).

The same thing happened when glasses for farsightedness were fitted onto the primates. The eyesight actually got worse over time, not better!

At the very best, wearing glasses is a compromise. In no way can glasses be considered a solution to vision problems. They are a crutch, and as we've seen, a very problematic one. And they are a hassle. Consider the associated problems that come with having to wear glasses...

- Forgetting where you put them
- Embarrassing reflections
- Having to change to sunglasses every time you go out in the sun
- Discomfort
- Glasses slipping down your nose
- Hassles when playing a sport
- Glasses fogging up

Your glasses will get dirty, they will scratch and will, at some stage, get stepped on. Wearing glasses will also negatively impact your peripheral vision. The frames tend to block your side vision. Wearing glasses may also require you to visit your eye doctor regularly to have glasses adjusted, as your eyes can get lazy from using the glasses too much. As a result, your vision can steadily decrease over time.

The frames of eyeglasses also have a tendency to lose their shape over time, especially when worn on a daily basis. This will require that you consult an eye doctor to have them adjusted.

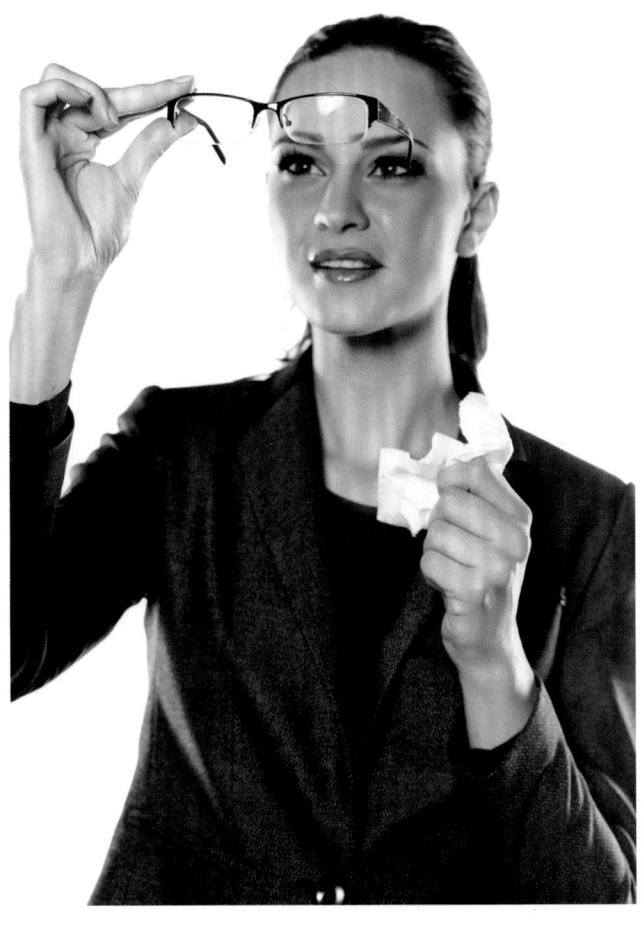

You may also decide to buy prescription sunglasses, which can be pretty expensive, for use in addition to your regular glasses. There are glasses that can turn from clear indoors to dark outdoors, but they cost an awful lot of money.

Then there is the weather. Glasses fog up in cold weather and make it very hard to see in the rain.

Even the most basic pair of glasses can cost around $400 – that's as much as many people's phones!

So why is a simple piece of plastic the same price as the miracle of technology that is your smartphone?

Eighty percent of glasses and sunglasses brands are controlled by a single company…

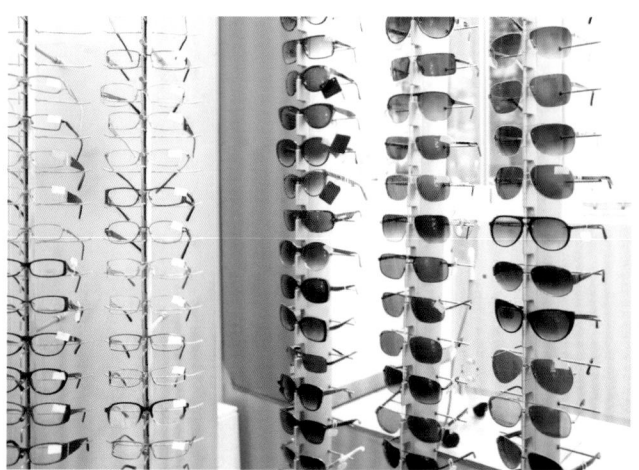

This gives them a virtual monopoly over the entire industry. Because they control both the luxury brands and the cheap brands, they can charge whatever they want for either.

Luxottica uses that power to drive up the price of glasses for everybody, charging as much as 20 times what they cost to produce.

It's not just prescription glasses.

Ray-Bans used to be bargain mass-market sunglasses worn by everyone. But in 1999, Luxottica bought the brand and raised the price to $150 per pair – 4X what they used to be!

Seventy percent of Luxottica's brands come from the exact same factory. And Luxottica owns almost all of the glasses stores that are out there. That means that the few brands that they don't own are forced to obey their demands.

When Oakley tried to dispute Luxottica's pricing, Luxottica retaliated by dropping Oakley glasses from all of their stores. Oakley's price collapsed – and Luxottica swooped in and bought them out.

Luxottica has so much power that, when a company didn't play by their rules, they took them to the brink of destruction – and then took over that company.

Luxottica also owns the second largest eye insurance company in America. That means that it is possible for your optometrist, your insurance company, the factory that makes your frames and the store that sells them to you to all be owned by the same company.

So, why isn't every pair of glasses out there labeled Luxottica?

Because Luxottica is selling you the illusion of choice.

The Problem with Contacts

If you thought glasses were bad for your eyes, get ready to be shocked.

Contact lenses are **even worse**.

The long-term effects of contact lens wear on the cornea may include:

- Changes in the thickness of the cornea
- Alterations to the curvature of the cornea

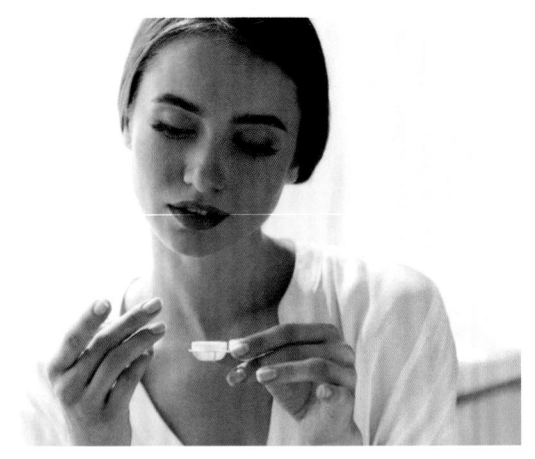

- A diminished level of epithelial oxygen uptake by the eye
- The formation of epithelial vacuoles and microcysts
- Diminished corneal sensitivity
- Photophobia
- Vision loss

A lot of study has gone into the effect of long-term use of contact lenses, with the above consequences being well documented. Similar results have been found between users of both hard and soft contact lenses. However, the more rigid edges of hard contact lenses do appear to generate a greater degree of trauma in the eye.

The bottom line appears to be that whenever a physical barrier is placed over the cornea, problems will occur. Not surprisingly, it is the cornea that is most adversely affected by contact lenses.

Eye Structure and Contacts

Prolonged use of soft hydrogel contacts actually changes the shape of the cornea. Specifically, it alters the thickness of the epithelial cells. It also increases the corneal curvature. This can be as much as 0.5 diopters more than normal. Long-term contact wear can also lead to an irregular and asymmetrical cornea.

All of this leads to chronic stress to the cornea.

Using hard contacts made from thick hydrogel is even worse than soft contacts. It can lead to warping of the cornea. However, studies have found that soft lenses lead to greater corneal steeping. A normal cornea is round, with even curvature like that of a sphere. With a steep cornea,

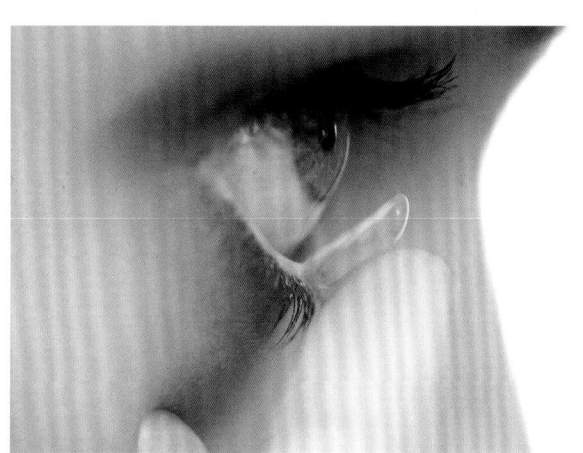

the curvature is irregular and too steep, like the narrow end of an egg. If the corneal shape is excessively steep, flat, or not completely round, it can cause nearsightedness, farsightedness or astigmatism.

Fortunately, many of the problems brought on by contact lens use are not irreversible. The uptake of epithelial oxygen returns to normal for most people about a month after they stop using contacts. The thickness of the epithelial cells should return to normal about a week after stopping the use of contacts.

But there are some effects that do not return to normal. Endothelial polymegethism will not revert back to its pre-contact lens level, even years after you stop wearing the contacts. The same goes for stromal thickness. It could also take up to three months for microcysts to disappear.

Hygiene and Contact Lenses

Putting your fingers into your eyes every day to put in and take out contacts turns out to be not such a good idea. Putting contacts in your eye is not a harmless act.

Researchers at NYU's Langone Medical Center found significant differences in the ecosystems of people who wear contact lenses and those who don't. In one study, they took swabs of hundreds of people's eye conjunctiva, which covers the white part of your eye. They found thousands of strains of bacteria in the different parts of the eye. But the people who wore contacts had more bacterial diversity in the skin beneath their eye and a higher amount of different types of bacteria on the surface of the eye itself (4).

In fact, the contact lens wearers had three times the usual proportion of such bacteria as...

- Methylobacterium
- Lactobacillus
- Pseudomonas bacteria

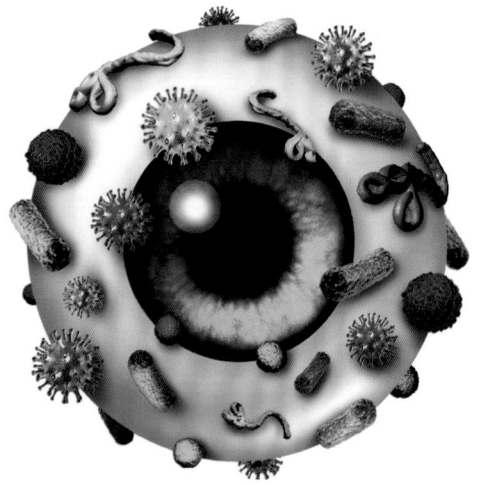

The bacteria on the surface of the eyes of the contact wearers looked more like the bacteria found on their skin when compared to the people who didn't wear contacts at all.

Whether this high concentration of bacteria in the eyes of contact lens wearers is because people keep touching their eyes with their dirty fingers, or if it is the lens itself that is changing the composition of the eye, researchers are unsure at this time.

What they *are* sure about is that wearers of contact lenses get more frequent eye infections. Since the 1950s, when soft contact lenses came onto the scene, corneal ulcers have increased at an alarming rate.

Corneal ulcers leave an open, nasty sore on the cornea. This is caused by bacterial, fungal or viral infections. The kind of bacteria that causes a corneal ulcer is found on the skin. This suggests that poor hand hygiene is to blame.

A study published in *Optometry and Vision Science* identified three specific behaviors that might lead to nasty infections:

- Not washing hands with soap and water before handling contacts
- Not letting the contact lens case air dry
- Using a contact case and a solution from different manufacturers (5) (6) (7)

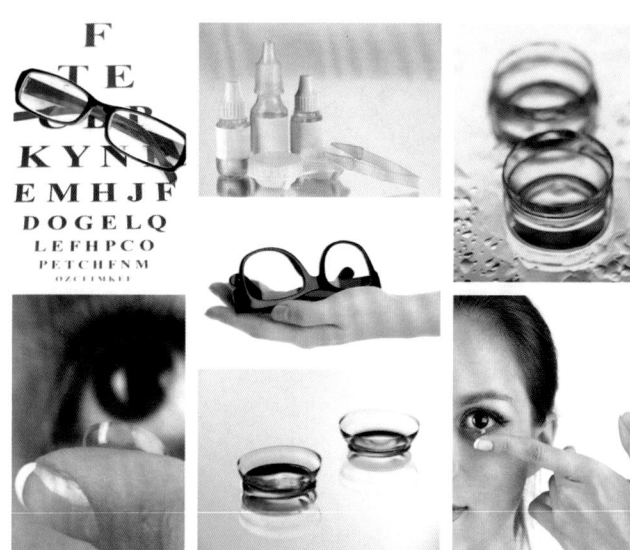

People who are too lazy to follow these guidelines do have the option of using contacts that have an antibacterial coating. A study that was published in Vision Science magazine involved testing a contact lens that was coated with melamine. Melamine fights microbes by inhibiting their growth. In this study, volunteers wore these contacts for a day with no major side effects (8) (9) (10).

Knowing that you have bacteria in your eye may sound scary. Yet, bacteria are everywhere in and on us. Not all of it is bad. Our microbiome is beneficial for our health.

However, some bacteria cause nasty infections. And the one area where you don't want nasty bacteria to run amuck is in your eyes (11).

Cleaning and storing contact lenses can be a hassle. It requires washing your hands first, taking the contact lenses out of your eyes, and cleaning them with a cleaning solution. Then, you have to replace the old solution in your lens case with new solution. Finally, you need to put your contacts into the new solution and in your lens case until you are ready to use them again (12).

The worst part of wearing contacts is actually putting them on. It is especially difficult if you tend to blink a lot or are not used to wearing contacts. Putting a foreign object into your eyes can make you automatically close your eyes (13).

For many people, wearing contacts never stops feeling uncomfortable.

CHAPTER FIVE

WHY SURGERY IS DEFINITELY NOT THE ANSWER

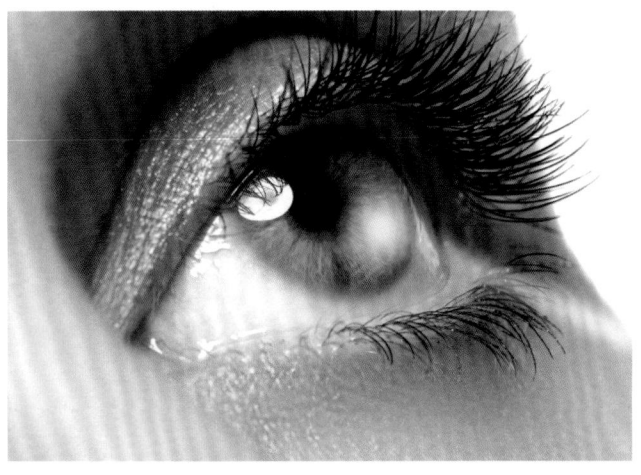

Surgical procedures that are designed to correct faulty vision are known as 'vision corrective surgery.' It is also called laser eye surgery. In the past decade, great strides have been made in this form of treatment.

The majority of types of vision corrective surgery involve changing the shape of the cornea. This enables the light coursing through the cornea to better focus on the retina.

These are the most common types of vision corrective surgery:

Laser In-Situ Keratomileusis (LASIK)

LASIK surgery is used to improve eyesight in nearsighted and farsighted people and in people with astigmatism. It involves reshaping the tissue under the cornea. This allows it to focus light properly into the eyes.

With LASIK surgery, the surgeon makes a flap in the outer part of the cornea in order to access the tissue under the cornea. A computer imaging procedure, known as wavefront technology, may also be used in conjunction with LASIK in order to create a detailed image of the cornea, which helps to guide the surgery.

Photorefractive Keratectomy (PRK)

This type of surgery is used to improve the eyesight of mildly to moderately nearsighted and farsighted people and those who have astigmatism. A laser beam is used by the eye surgeon to reshape the cornea. The laser projects a beam of pulsing UV light that is directed into the corneal surface of the eye.

Laser Epithelial Keratomileusis (LASEK)

This type of surgery is a variant of PRK. The eye surgeon creates an epithelial flap, and then the epithelial cells are loosened by an alcohol solution. A laser is then used to reshape the cornea. Afterwards, the flap is replaced with a soft contact lens to secure the eye while it heals. This kind of procedure is used to correct the vision of nearsighted and farsighted people, and those with astigmatism.

Automated Lamellar Keratoplasty (ALK)

This type of surgery is for treating people with extreme nearsightedness and those with minimal degrees of hyperopia (farsightedness). Similar to LASIK, a flap is made in the cornea to allow the surgeon to reach the tissue under the cornea. The difference is that ALK does not require a laser. Rather, one more incision is created on the outer part of the cornea to reshape it.

Refractive Lens Exchange (RLE)

This type of surgery is also known as clear lens extraction. It is quite similar to cataract surgery. It involves making a small incision at the edge of the cornea to replace the natural lens with a silicone or plastic lens.

Refractive lens exchange is used in correcting severe farsightedness or nearsightedness.

This type of surgery may be appropriate for those with thin corneas, dry eyes or other corneal problems. However, other types of procedures are needed to correct problems with astigmatism.

Epi-Lasik

This type of surgery is similar to PRK. A very thin layer is separated from the cornea and is either left off or replaced. The cornea is then either left off or replaced. The cornea is then reshaped, and the area is protected with a soft contact lens while it is healing.

Presbyopic Lens Exchange (PRELEX)

Presbyopia is a condition wherein the eye's lens is no longer flexible. It then becomes more difficult for the eye to focus on nearby objects. Presbyopic lens exchange (PRELEX) is a type of eye surgery where a multi-focus lens is implanted for the correction of presbyopia.

Intracorneal Ring Segments (INTACS)

The intracorneal ring (ICR) segments procedure involves creating a small incision in the cornea and then placing two crescent-shaped plastic rings at the outer edge of the cornea. These two rings reshape the cornea, flattening it to change the way light rays focus on the retina.

This type of procedure was originally used to treat mild nearsightedness. However, it was replaced by laser-based procedures. Occasionally, an irregular astigmatism associated with Keratoconus is a condition wherein there is thinning and irregularity in the cornea that could lead to loss of eyesight.

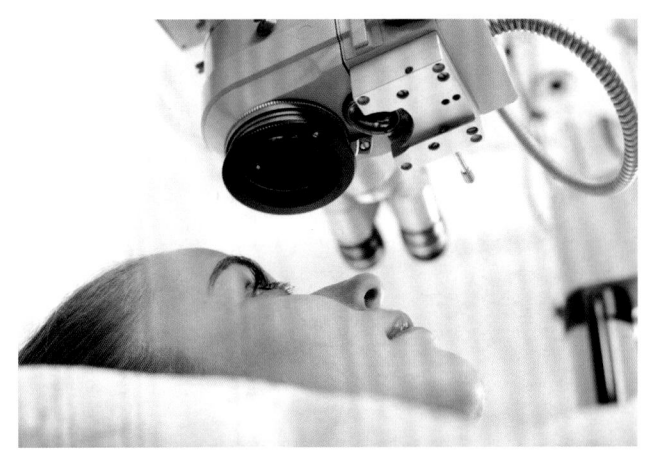

Phakic Intraocular Lens Implants

Patients who are too nearsighted to have LASIK and PRK procedures can benefit from phakic implants that are inserted through a small incision at the edge of the cornea. It is then attached to the iris and inserted behind the pupil. The difference between phakic implants and RLE is that the eye's natural lens is left in its original place.

Astigmatic Keratotomy (AK)

People who have an astigmatism have football shaped corneas. Astigmatic keratotomy (AK) is a surgical procedure that is used to correct the vision of people with an astigmatism. However, a laser is not used in this procedure. Rather, the surgeon creates a single or double incision at the area of the cornea where it is most steep. Those two incisions enable the cornea to be more relaxed and become rounder in shape. It is possible to use this procedure by itself or in conjunction with some other type of laser eye surgery.

Radial Keratotomy (RK)

Radial keratotomy is a type of procedure that used to be one of the most commonly used procedures for correcting nearsightedness. However, there is an increasing number of successful laser eye surgeries that have been developed. These have made radial keratotomy pretty much redundant, and it is rarely used these days.

The Problems with Eye Surgery

LASIK surgery is advertised as a nearly miraculous surgical method of vision correction. It is estimated that since LASIK became widely available in the late 1990s, some 18 million patients have undergone laser eye surgery.

However, many thousands of those patients have experienced serious complications. These include everything from blurred vision to blindness.

The first step of a LASIK procedure involves taking a low dose of valium to help you stay relaxed during surgery. You then sign a patient consent form. In this form, you state that you understand the risks involved in the procedure and give up your rights to sue if things go wrong.

The procedure itself takes about 10 minutes. There are various ways of doing it depending on your specific eye condition. One involves placing a suction device onto the eye. This places an enormous amount of suction pressure on the eye. A microkeratome plate then makes a flap parallel to the surface of the eye, which leaves a hinge on the cornea. The flap is then folded over. Your eye is then shot with a laser.

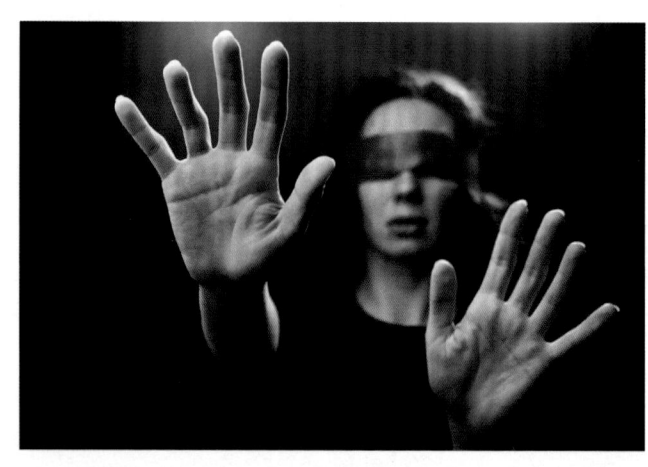

Then they move on to the other eye.

Though costs can vary from $1500 - $5000 per eye, it is an enormously expensive 10 minutes.

After the procedure, you will have the sensation of thousands of needles sticking into your eyeballs. Phantom sensations of this feeling will persist indefinitely.

Many people's eyes do not heal properly post-procedure. They won't be able to put in contacts or wear glasses in the year following the procedure. Despite being told that the procedure would be great and would restore 20/20 vision, they find out that everything they were promised was a lie. For many people, their vision actually gets worse.

Despite this, the LASIK industry reports a great success rate. Their research claims that it is as high as 95%. That statistic is completely and utterly out of touch with reality.

In fact, Maurice Waxler, the doctor who originally approved LASIK surgery for the FDA, is now a prominent opponent of the procedure. After researching the data relating to patient experiences, Dr. Waxler saw that he had been duped by the ophthalmologists who were pushing the LASIK surgery wagon.

In order to get LASIK surgery through the FDA process, the doctors put adverse effects from the procedure into the wrong column. Things such as permanent halos, dry eye, double vision and blindness were placed in a column marked *temporary side effects* in order to get it approved. It wasn't until some 15 years later that this was brought to his attention by a group of thousands of people who had been through the nightmare of LASIK surgery.

Since 2009, Dr. Waxler has been petitioning the FDA to have LASIK surgery stopped. He has even referred to the surgeons who perform LASIK as charlatans, saying that they are not even doctors. Doctors have taken a Hippocratic oath to help people who are sick to become healthy. Yet those who perform LASIK surgery are actually taking a healthy eye and making it a sick and diseased eye. Dr. Waxler is now pushing for a criminal investigation into those doctors who have been falsifying and fabricating the information upon which FDA approval was granted.

How many people are affected by this scam?

Statistics tell us that around 18 million people in the US alone have had the operation. Some 3.4 million of those eyes have permanent damage. One result of the surgery is dry eye, which is why there has been a great increase in people with this condition since the turn of the century. It is also why there have been so many dry eyedrop commercials on TV in recent years. What the ads don't tell you is that the root of the dry eye problem is the wonderful panacea treatment of laser eye surgery.

In fact, many eye drop bottles say on the label that it is 'For LASIK dry eye.'

After LASIK surgery, your eye is not able to produce a tear film to keep it healthy and moist. When the eye is slashed open, you are cutting into vital corneal nerves that are meant to tell the brain to send tears to the eyes.

Not only are people not adequately informed about the dangers of LASIK

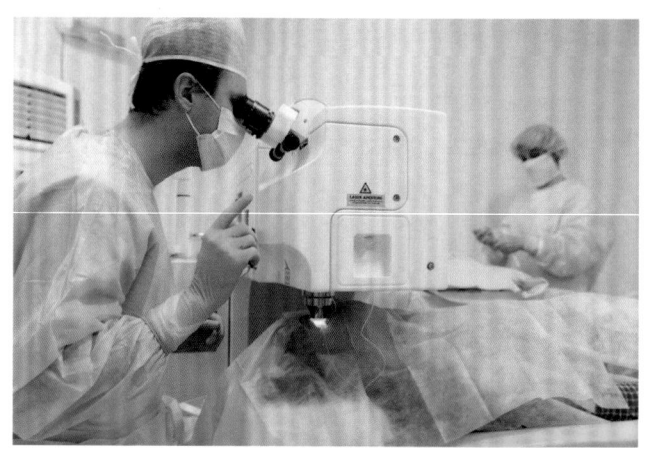

surgery, they are actually tricked with deceptive advertising. The FDA requires that any advertising for LASIK treatments, be it on TV, the Internet, radio, or by way of brochures, list all of the possible adverse effects. Yet the LASIK industry has ignored this requirement – and the FDA has been totally negligent in enforcing compliance.

The result is that the public has been duped into believing that this procedure was safe. They know that it was approved by the FDA. However, they aren't aware that Dr. Waxler, who gave the FDA the green light on LASIK, is now adamantly opposed to the procedure. That's because he was deceived, and is now wanting a criminal investigation into the whole sordid affair.

There is very little recourse when you experience post-LASIK problems. I have not heard of a single person who has been cured of dry eye following the procedure. In fact, from year to year, the problems actually get worse.

Many people have spent many times the already outrageous cost of the initial surgery traveling the globe, looking for a way to correct the myriad problems that LASIK surgery has caused for their eyes – to no avail. They have tried everything from saline washes to different types of glasses with custom-made lenses. And contacts aren't even worth trying because, once you've had LASIK surgery, your eyes won't be able to produce enough tear film to allow you to wear them.

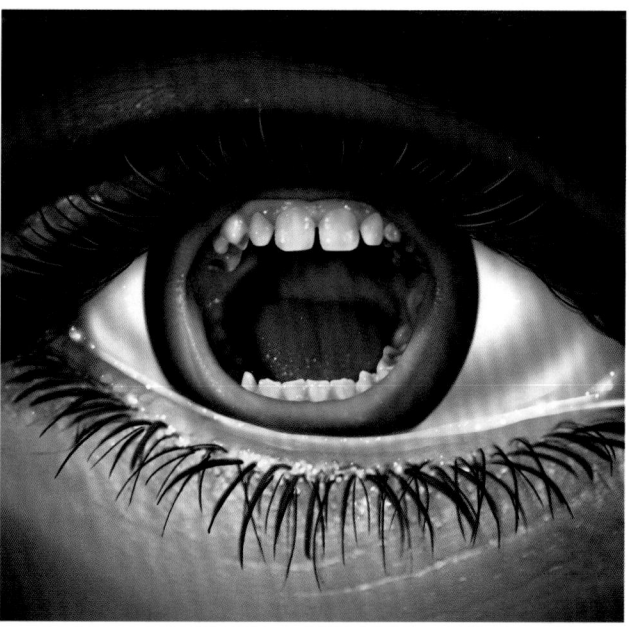

The Frightening Effects of LASIK that Have Been Hidden from You

- LASIK causes dry eye – symptoms of dry eye include burning, pinprick, foreign body sensation, scratchiness, soreness and the eyelid sticking to the eyeball (14).

- LASIK results in LOSS of visual quality – LASIK patients have more trouble seeing detail in dim light (loss of contrast sensitivity) an experience and increase in visual symptoms at night (halos, starbursts, glare, double vision, ghosting) (15).

- LASIK permanently damages the cornea – the cornea is not capable of complete healing after LASIK. In fact, it is permanently weakened. The collagen bands of the cornea provide its full form and strength. LASIK severs these collagen bands and thins the cornea (16).

- LASIK results in long-term consequences – LASIK affects the accuracy of intraocular pressure measurements, exposing patients to risk of vision loss from undiagnosed glaucoma.

Another study found that people who have undergone LASIK have cataract surgery six years sooner than people who have not had LASIK (17).

- LASIK surgery may produce serious complications down the line – the medical literature contains numerous reports of late-onset LASIK complications, such as loss of the cornea due to biomechanical instability, inflammation resulting in corneal haze, flap dislocation, epithelial ingrowth, and retinal detachment.

Complications may emerge weeks, months or even years after seemingly successful LASIK surgery.

- LASIK does not eliminate the need for glasses – it does not eliminate the need for reading glasses after the age of 40 and studies show that visual outcomes of LASIK decline over time.
- LASIK's true rate of complications is unknown – the FDA allowed laser manufacturers to hide complications reported by LASIK patients in clinical trials by classifying dry eyes and night vision impairment as symptoms instead of complications.
- Post LASIK rehabilitation options are limited – LASIK is irreversible, and treatment options for complications are extremely limited (18).

So now you know.

The panacea of eye surgery had turned out to be a scam. Not only is it not the solution to your vision problems…

It is dangerous to your eyes.

Never let a surgeon with a scalpel get anywhere near your eyes.

So, if glasses and contact lenses are nothing more than a problematic crutch and laser surgery is a nightmare, what are we left with?

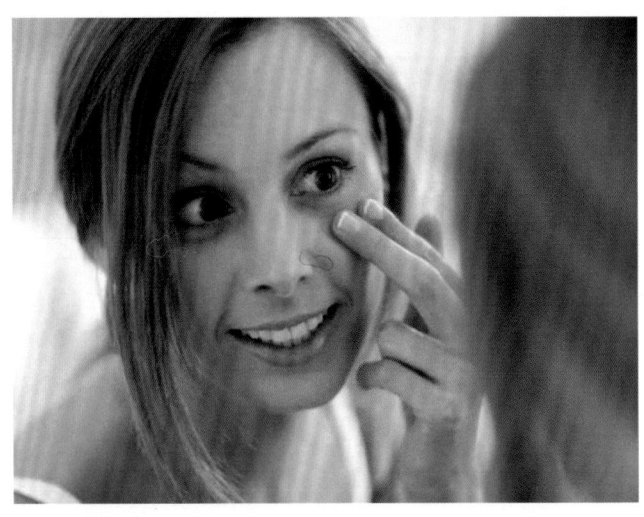

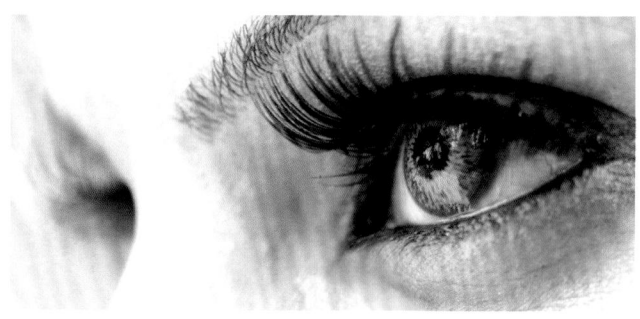

The real solution to achieving 20/20 vision is actually the simplest – and the most inexpensive.

So, why haven't you heard of it?

Well, just flick back over this chapter and you'll get an idea of the obscene amounts of money that the eye industry has been making.

After all, you've been lied to and manipulated your entire life into believing that corrective lenses or miracle surgery are your only options. Because, of course, the $36 billion optometry industry will never tell you that there's a quick, easy and natural way to restore your vision.

If they did, nobody would ever need a pair of glasses again!

Chapter SIX

WHAT'S THE DEAL WITH EYE EXERCISES?

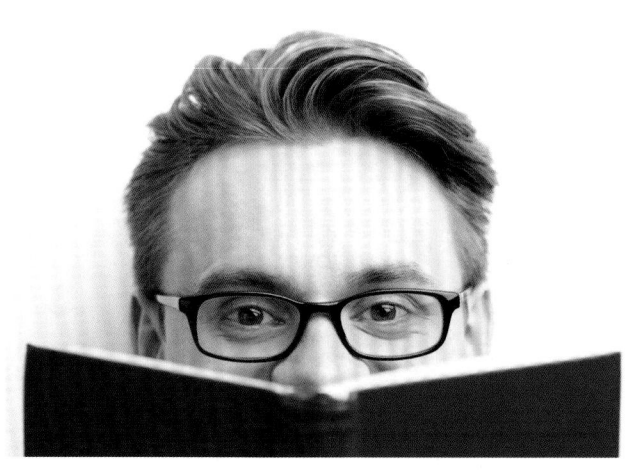

Just go on YouTube, and you'll find a ton of videos on eye exercises that are supposed to give you clearer vision.

So, can exercises really improve your eyesight?

Well, let's take a moment to find out what these exercises are and where they came from.

People have held the belief that certain exercises of the eyes can improve vision for thousands of years. However, it wasn't until the publication of a book by a doctor named William Horatio Bates in 1920 that the practice was formalized in the Western world.

The book that Dr. Bates wrote was called

The Cure of Imperfect Eyesight by Treatment Without Glasses

Three years earlier, Bates had joined forces with a popular strength and physical culture promoter and publisher named Bernarr McFadden. McFadden had a magazine called *Physical Culture*. Through the magazine, the pair offered an eye treatment course that promised amazing results with some basic exercises. The course was a success, and it led to Bates being acknowledged as an authority in vision restoration though he was not trained in that field.

When Bates published his book in 1920, he enjoyed even greater success. Inevitably, many other books, pamphlets and courses soon followed, with others eager to capitalize on his success. Most of them told their readers to throw away their glasses and start using the 'Bates' method immediately.

However, the whole basis of the Bates method was built upon a fallacy. He asserted that errors of refraction are not the result of the basic shape of the eyeball, but rather to weakness in the muscles on the outside of the eyeball. And, of course, all that weak muscles needed was exercise.

According to Bates, every eye problem that was experienced by every person in the world was essentially a product of eye strain or nervous tension. When you learn to completely relax your eyes, he taught, your vision will increase dramatically. He further stated that glasses actually make your eyes worse. Sunglasses, according to Bates, were even more damaging.

Bates promoted his method as the ultimate solution for such problems as...

- Nearsightedness
- Farsightedness
- Astigmatism
- Presbyopia
- Cataracts
- Eye infections
- Glaucoma
- Macular Degeneration

The exercises that Bates advocated included palming, which is when you cover your eyes, focus on blackness, and rapidly shift your eyes from side to side. It should seem pretty obvious to you that these types of actions are going to do absolutely nothing when it comes to correcting the problems listed above.

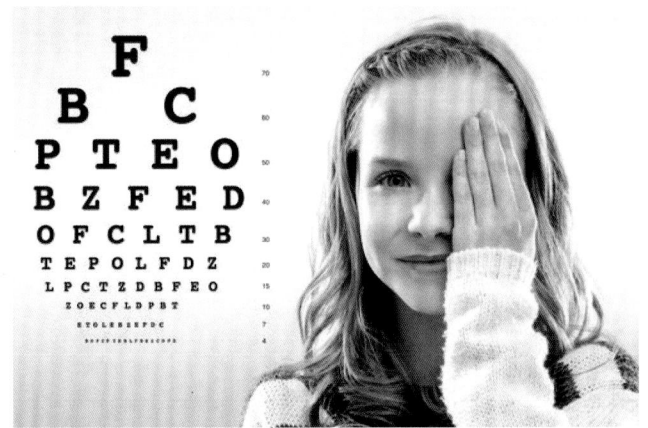

In fact, the types of claims that Bates made in his book and other advertising were so outrageous that, in 1929, the

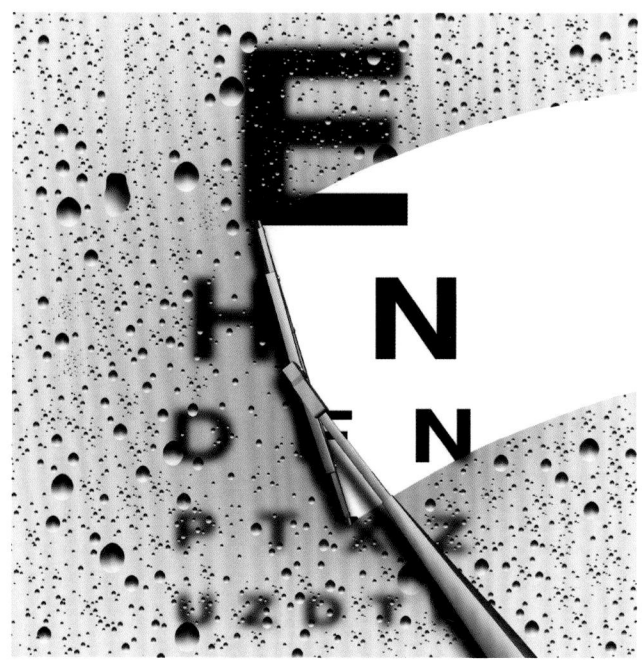

Federal Trade Commission filed a complaint claiming that his advertising was false and misleading.

William Horatio Bates died in 1931. However, that was not the end of his crazy eye exercise ideas. His wife, Emily, was to continue his legacy. Along with Dr. Harold M. Peppard, she took the eye exercise concept to new levels.

In 1940, the original book was re-released as *Better Eyesight Without Glasses*. A version of that book is still in print today. One of the treatments that the book advocates is sun treatment, which involves focusing the whites of the eyes on the sun.

The first real critique of the Bates method came in the 1950s with the publication of a book by a prominent optometrist named Philip Pollack.

Today, the vast majority of educated people see the Bates method for what it is: a scam.

However, eye exercises have made a comeback because of the wide dissemination available on the Internet. The new advocates of the Bates method are known as Vision Therapists.

Vision Therapists believe that eyesight can be improved with exercises, just like Bates. The difference, however, is that Vision Therapists advocate what are called 'active exercises.' These include the following methods:

- Eye focusing
- Eye pointing
- Eye movement skills

The actual exercises included such things as eye-hand coordination drills, watching blinking lights, bouncing up and down on a trampoline and even sleeping in a certain position.

The advocates of Vision Therapy don't just claim that it can eliminate the need for glasses or contacts. They state that it can also improve a person's education, boost their athletic performance and up their IQ level. They even claim that it can prevent juvenile delinquency.

Of course, there is absolutely no scientific backing for these claims. In fact, just the opposite.

In 2009, the UK's College of Optometrists undertook a large-scale investigation of 10 controversial Vision Therapy treatments. Here is what they concluded...

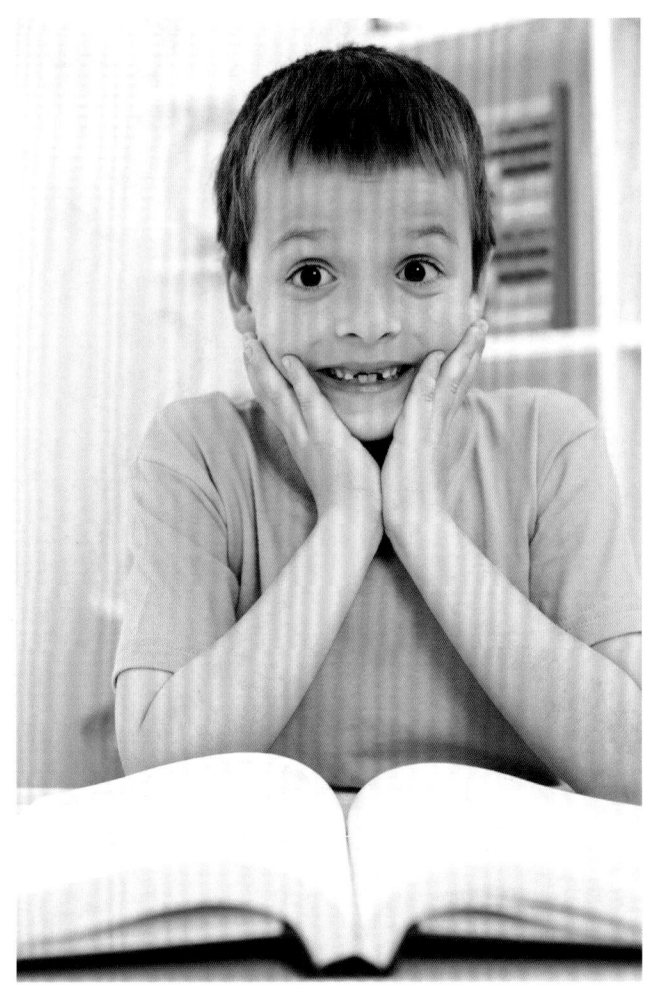

There is a continued paucity of controlled trials in the literature to support behavioral optometry approaches. Although there are areas where the available evidence is consistent with claims made by behavioral optometrists (most notably in relation to the treatment of convergence insufficiency, the use of yoked prisms in neurological patients, and in vision rehabilitation after brain disease / injury) a large majority of behavioral management approaches are not evidence based, and thus cannot be advocated (19).

The key premise behind the Vision Therapy approach is that problems with eyesight are the result of learned or environmental factors. They can, therefore, be corrected with eye training. One result of the proliferation of these ideas is that dyslexia can be corrected with Vision Therapy.

Many people think that dyslexia is a problem of the eyes. It is not. It is a reading disorder, stemming from the brain's inability to interpret the sound of spoken words or to process language information rapidly. Despite this, thousands of teachers continue to send dyslexic children to vision therapy training.

What About Iridology?

Iridology is based on the idea that every part of the eye represents a corresponding part of the body. As a result, the health of the various parts of the body can be determined by the color, texture and pigmentation of various pigments in the eye. Iridologists then treat the perceived ailment with minerals, herbs and vitamins.

Two large studies tested the ability of iridologists to use the eyes as the 'television screen' to the body. In these studies, eight prominent iridologists were unable to tell the difference between patients who had kidney and gallbladder complaints and those who were healthy by looking into their eyes (20) (21).

This is hardly surprising, as there is no scientific evidence that the eyes represent the various organs of the body.

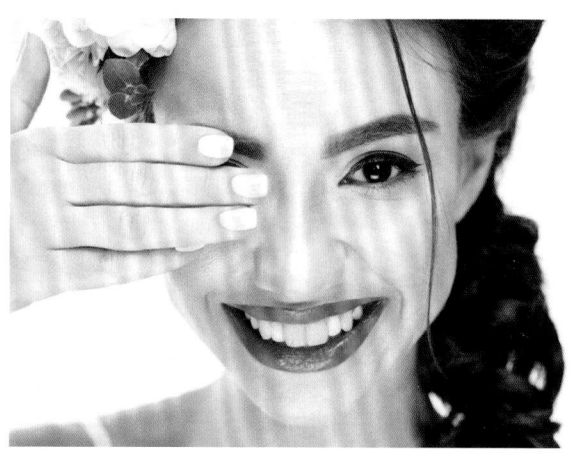

Palming Can Be Helpful

Although the vast majority of eye exercises will not do a thing to improve your vision, there is one technique that is beneficial. This technique is not for vision correction, but to relax the eyes and the nervous system.

It is called **PALMING**.

To begin palming, rub your hands together to get them warm and relaxed. Allow your fingers to interlace to get the entire surface of the hands warm.

Now, take the palm of one hand and gently cover the eye. Your goal is to block out light. Then, bring up the other hand to cover the other eye. You will find that by crossing the hands, you are more effective at blocking out the light.

Be sure not to press on the eyeball. You want to cover the eye so that the palms cup around the eyeball. Check for light coming through – you want to shut out as much as possible.

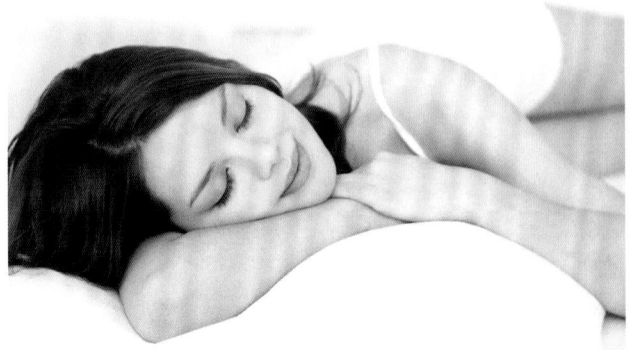

Now breathe deeply and tune into the black areas. Sense the black visual areas and feel your bones. Drop your head and elbows to relax the shoulders. If you're sitting at a desk, lean your elbows on the desk.

Continue breathing and tuning into the black areas. This allows all of the muscles around the eyes to relax. Notice the sounds around you.

Do this exercise for as long as it feels comfortable for you. A good 30 seconds to a minute is very refreshing. With practice, the black will get blacker.

When finished, keep your eyes closed as you remove your hands. With eyes still closed, notice the light. Having periods of darkness and light like this is recharging for the brain. Now, slowly open your eyes. Blinking is a very good way to move the fluids around your eyes.

You can practice this standing or sitting. The best way to do it, however, is lying down.

If you have trouble sleeping, try doing this palming exercise in bed at night. It is a wonderful aid to help you drift off. It will calm down your whole system, relieving anxiety.

To conclude this chapter on eye exercises, let's consider basic eye biology. The distance between the front of your eye (cornea) and the back of the eye (retina) is called the axial length. If that axial length is too great, you will have nearsightedness (myopia). You will only have good vision for close objects. What is far away will be blurry. If your axial length is too short, you will have farsightedness (hyperopia). In this case, you will be able to see far away but not up close.

Now, you can do as many exercises as you want, for as long as you want, but you cannot actually change the length of the eyeball. This is a bit like working out your arms. You can make your biceps, triceps and forearms bigger, but can you actually increase the length of your arm?

NO.

Apart from the fact that they don't work, eye exercises are also not sustainable. Nobody wants to have to perform monotonous and repetitive eye exercises every day of their life in order to have clear vision.

So, forget about those useless YouTube videos and monotonous eye exercises. They hold no benefit for your eyesight.

Having taken care of the things that won't correct your vision…

- Glasses
- Contact Lenses
- Laser eye surgery
- Eye exercises

…we can now focus on the things that will.

CHAPTER **SEVEN**

SIX VISION HABITS YOU CAN ADOPT TODAY

In this chapter, you will discover a half-dozen vision habits that will reduce the mental and physical strain that could affect your eyesight. Making these habits second nature will help keep your vision as clear, sharp and relaxed as it can be.

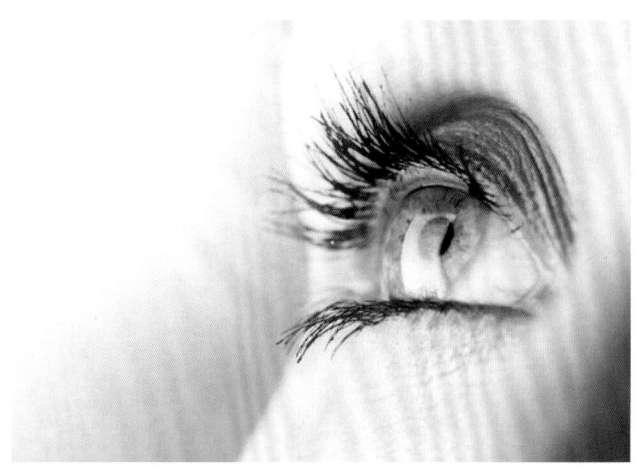

Habit No.1: Blink Regularly

Blinking cleanses and lubricates the eyes. When there is no tension, your eyes blink 10 - 12 times every minute, or about once every five seconds. But people who do not see clearly tend to stare and unconsciously hold their eyes open. This causes strain, as well as the feeling of dry and tired eyes.

Consciously remind yourself to blink every five seconds. Of course, you don't want to go through the day with a stopwatch, but the more conscious you are of blinking regularly, the better it is for your eyes.

The eyelid is the only part of the body that is controlled by just one muscle. Any other movement usually involves two muscles – one that contracts and one that stretches to make the movement. Your eyelid is controlled by only one muscle. Having proper relaxation in that muscle can promote relaxation throughout the entire body. That's why you often hear hypnotists using the phrase 'your eyes are becoming heavy' as a way to get the subject to relax.

A blinking exercise that you can practice throughout the day is called

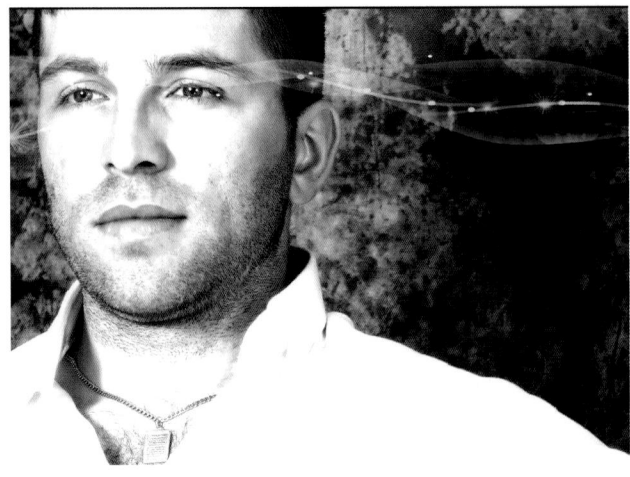

and a tense style of concentration.

In order to relieve this strain on your eyes, always remind yourself to be aware of your peripheral vision. Be aware of everything as you are looking at one point.

Habit No. 3: Keep Your Eyes Moving and Change Your Focus

Keeping your eyes moving and changing your focus is the most direct way to break the staring habit. Normally, the eye moves slightly about 50 - 60 times every second. It is constantly changing what it is looking at. This subtle movement is vital for clear vision. Staring and not consciously moving your eyes interferes with it.

When you remember to frequently change your focus, you will unlock the tension in your visual system. Your eyes will then become more relaxed. The key is to keep your eyes moving. When you're on the computer, make sure that you look up and focus on something in the distance at least once every 3 - 5 minutes.

'flutter blinking.' To do this, blink your eyes lightly and rapidly 10 - 20 times. Don't strain or squeeze your eyes shut, and relax your face as you blink. Then, close your eyes and relax. Repeat this 2 - 3 times.

Flutter blinking will help keep your eyes moist, relaxed and free of strain.

Habit No. 2: Use Your Peripheral Vision

All day long, as we are focusing on an object, other objects come into our view from the sides of our eyes. People with poor vision have so trained their minds to intently focus on just one thing that they block out their peripheral awareness. In a sense, they are putting on blinders. This breeds mental fatigue

Habit No. 4: Rest Your Eyes

Spend a minimum of 15 minutes every day in the outdoors where you have exposure to the sun. The kind of indoor lighting that you use is also important. Dr. John Ott, pioneer in the field of photobiology, which is the study of how different kinds of light affect living organisms, developed an indoor light that is the most complete substitute for sunlight. It is called Vita Lite and it easily replaces any standard fluorescent light. Studies have shown that using the Vita Lite increases see-ability, reduces glare and eyestrain, and improves visual acuity.

Your eyes are rested by total darkness. The best way to rest your eyes is to close them and place your cupped hand over your closed eyes, as described on page 60. When you do this regularly, you will be surprised at how refreshed you feel when you're done.

Habit No. 5: Breathe Deeply and Regularly

Breathing deeply and regularly helps to improve vision. It will keep your body more relaxed, help you concentrate for longer periods of time, and eliminate eyestrain and fatigue.

How to Do It

Stand or sit comfortably. Now, take in a long, deep breath through your nose until the lungs are completely full and your chest is inflated. Hold this breath for a full five seconds. Now, allow the breath to slowly leave your body. Be thinking about expanding and compressing the diaphragm (the muscle that expands and contracts your lungs), as if it were an accordion, on every inward and outward breath.

The Power of Nasal Breathing

Learning to breathe through your nose will make you a far more effective in-taker of oxygen. When you inhale through the nose, you will be taking the air more deeply into your diaphragm.

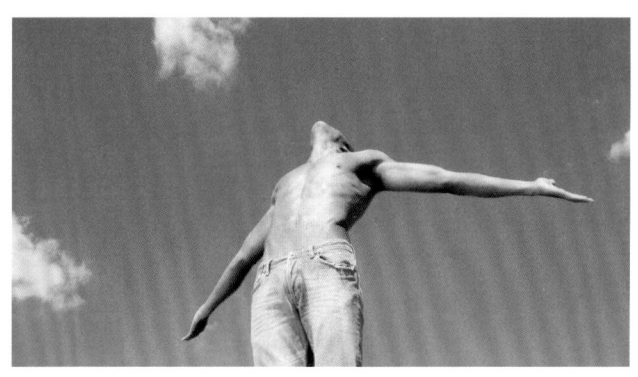

Try it right now, and you will be able to feel your diaphragm expanding. This expansion puts downward pressure on your abdomen. This has the flow-in effect of pushing air into the lungs and enhancing the circulation of blood and nutrients. This form of breathing is also more relaxing than mouth breathing.

Test Yourself: Breathe 100

Take in 100 nasal breaths in a row. Exhale through your mouth each time. Next, focus on breathing in with just your right nostril. Breathe out through your left. After 100 breaths, swap sides. As a final nasal challenge, breathe in 100 times, holding for 10 seconds after each breath.

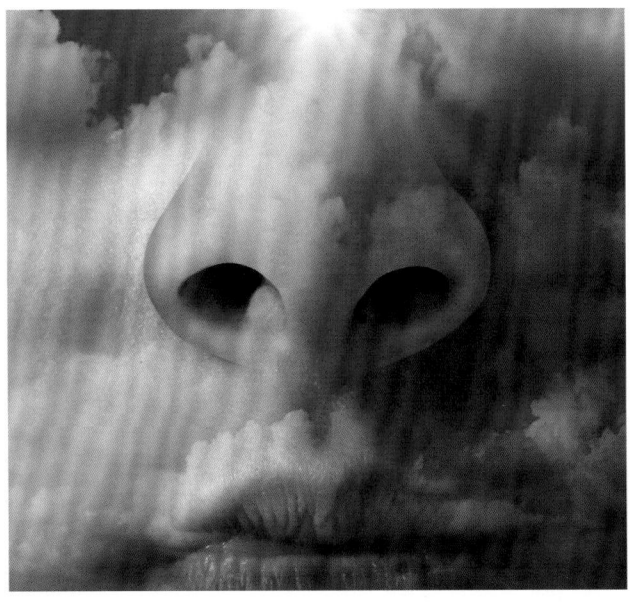

Sub-10: Your Breathing Goal

When you are breathing optimally, you will be taking in no more than 10 breaths a minute, and ideally just seven or eight. Your goal is to achieve as many sub-10 breath minutes as possible in your day.

Breathing Exercise

The breathing method just outlined will allow you to dramatically improve the amount of oxygen that comes into your body. That's great moving forward. However, you still have to contend with a whole lifetime of ineffective breathing. The following breathing exercise will allow you to strengthen and maintain power in your lungs.

Do this exercise first thing in the morning upon waking and again in midafternoon (it will provide a caffeine-free way of overcoming the 3 o'clock slump!).

Step One: Get comfortable, either standing or sitting.

Step Two: Breathe in through the nose for five seconds. Feel your stomach pushing out as the energy-giving oxygen fills your lungs.

Step Three: Hold for 20 seconds. Feel the oxygen circulating around your body as it gives life to your trillions of cells.

Step Four: Repeat this process four more times.

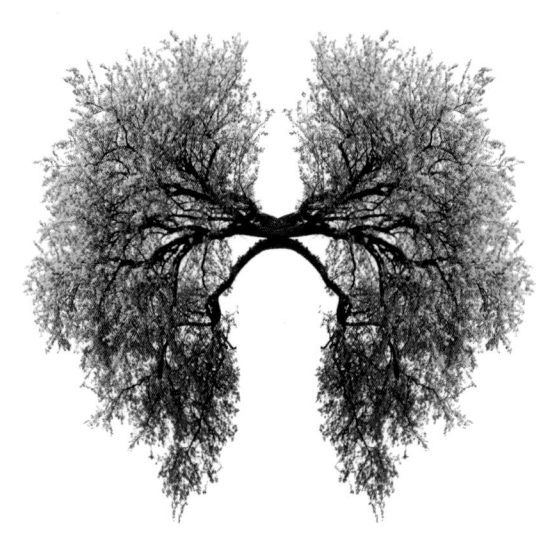

When performing lung exercises, it is important to focus on inflating the lungs upward and outward, rather than downward. Imagine that the intake of oxygen is about to lift you up and carry you skyward.

CHAPTER EIGHT

THE WISDOM OF THE ABORIGINE

Australia is home to many indigenous populations. There are, in fact, more than 400 distinct tribes. Aboriginal tribes are often grouped together and referred to as Aborigines. Legally, however, they are referred to as 'Aboriginals and Torres Strait Islanders.' Recent scientific studies have shown that Aboriginals may have left Africa up to 75,000 years ago. They would, therefore, represent one of the oldest continuous nations outside of Africa.

For centuries, these people thrived in Australia, normally in nomadic societies. They developed distinct tools, such as the boomerang, used for hunting, and the didgeridoo, a musical instrument that is still popular today. There are still legends and oral traditions that are referred to as 'dreaming.' These help explain their way of life and the world around them.

By the time the Europeans first established a colony in Australia in 1788, native populations were thought

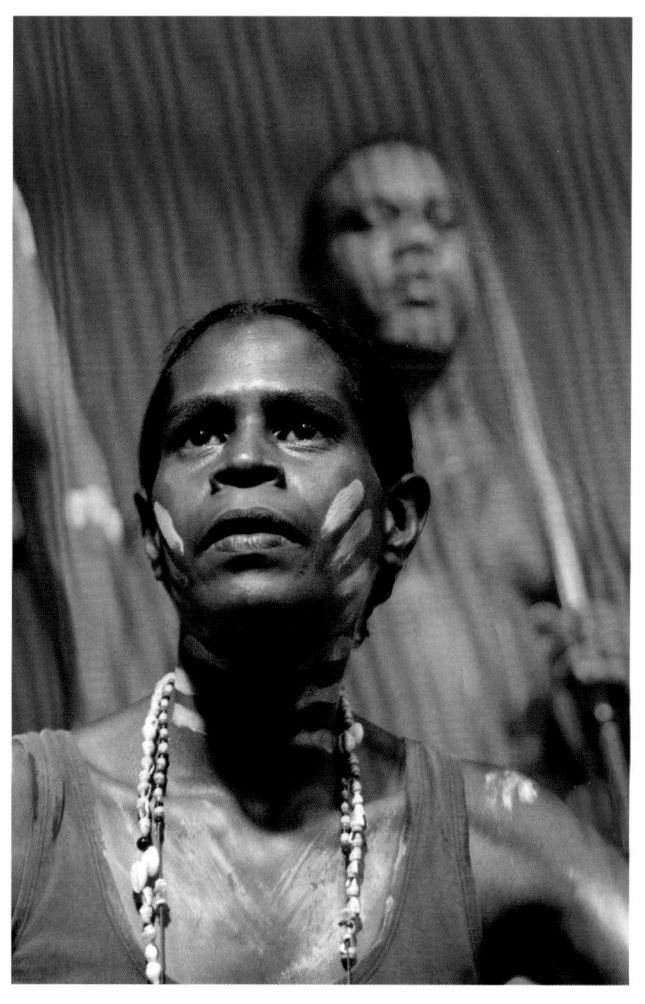

to number around 300,000. There were about 300 different languages spoken.

With the colonization of Australia, new diseases, violent racism and oppressive language policies devastated many of the original societies. Currently,

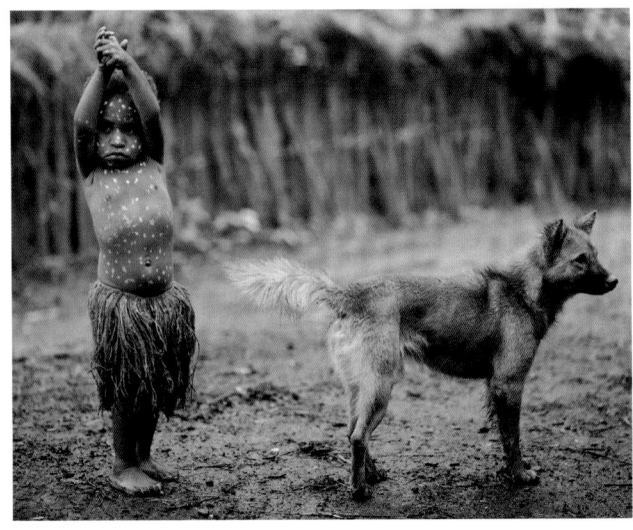

Aboriginal people account for just 3% of the Australian population. About 75 original languages still remain.

Until several decades ago, Aboriginals and Torres Strait Islanders faced extreme racism and government encroachment on their way of life. Many were not given Australian citizenship or Federal subsidies until the mid-twentieth century. Also during that time, the Australian government supported forcibly taking Aboriginal children from their parents. These would become known as the 'Stolen Generation.'

Well, that's all very interesting, you may be saying, but what has it got to do with improving your eyesight?

You're about to find out.

But to do so, I need to relate my personal journey.

I'm a retired Sergeant in the United States Marine Corps.

I've spent my entire adult life in battle, yet my experience of combat didn't prepare me for the hopelessness I felt when my beloved wife, Lindsay, faced an unseen enemy that was threatening to destroy her vision from the inside out.

Now, I'd built a reputation as a 'take charge' kinda guy, but I felt completely powerless as I witnessed the joy evaporating from my wife's being…

The light was going out of her eyes.

Thoughts raced through her mind, as she imagined the bleakest of futures.

No longer being able to see the smiles on her children's faces… the beautiful color of their eyes…

Or enjoy the sight of them growing up and becoming adults…

And then there were the simple things, like reading a book…

Watching her favorite TV shows…

Driving a car…

Or even seeing her own face in the mirror…

Her entire world was about to be plunged into endless darkness.

As the realization set in, Lindsay looked at me and broke down in tears.

I felt absolutely useless.

I so desperately wanted to solve this – to remove the burden.

But what could I do?

Day by day, Lindsay's vision got worse. Within two weeks, she was seriously struggling just to see me.

She hated the fact that she was losing her independence, and was scared about the future.

She talked about moving into an assisted living care home because she didn't want to be a burden on me or the kids.

As the days and weeks wore on, Lindsay became more and more depressed.

And then came the phone call.

It was my Staff Sergeant, telling me that I was to join a team of US Marines on a joint training exercise in the Australian Outback.

It was designed to improve surveillance techniques, and we were to work alongside Australia's North West Mobile Force, otherwise known as the NORFORCE Unit, a specialist

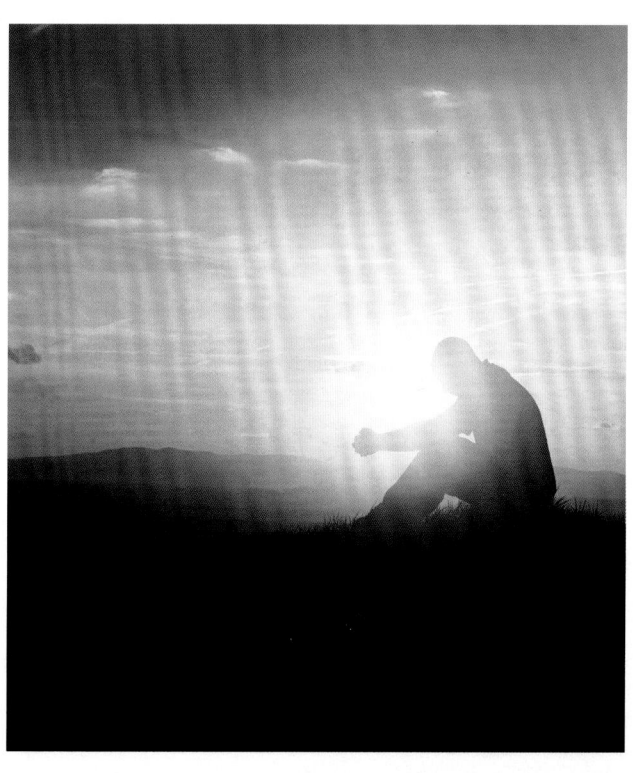

surveillance team made up of Aboriginal reservists who patrol the Outback in search of drug smugglers, human traffickers, asylum seekers and illegal foreign fishing vessels.

With Lindsay's condition, the timing couldn't have been worse – or so I thought.

But unable to do anything about it, I set off for Australia, leaving my mother-in-law and brother in charge of Lindsay's safety.

I hated leaving her – but as it turned out, the NORFORCE Unit would provide the answer to my prayers – and in the strangest of ways.

You see, on the third day of the training exercise, nine Marines, including myself, were teamed with an Aboriginal soldier called Bunji.

We were in camouflage, and Bunji was teaching us some old Aboriginal surveillance techniques, when he suddenly stopped dead in his tracks.

'See that?' he said, looking towards the water.

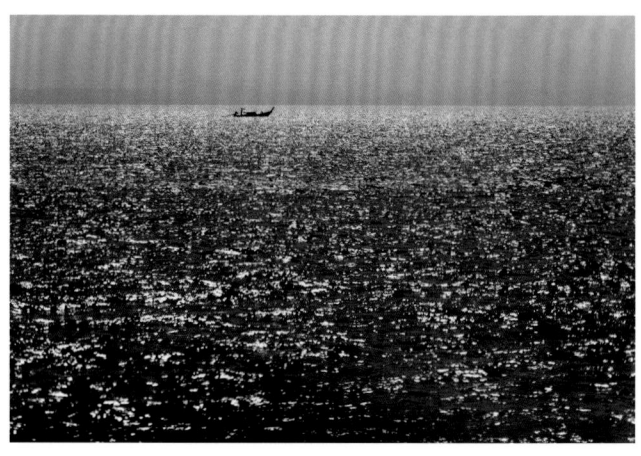

'See what?' I said.

None of us could see a thing.

'It's a vessel,' he replied.

I grabbed my binoculars and peered through them.

And there it was.

A small boat way off in the distance.

I could barely see it even with binoculars in front of my eyes, and I couldn't understand how the heck Bunji had seen it.

It was like spotting a grain of rice in the middle of a farmer's field.

He radioed his unit and within minutes, a 12-man team of NORFORCE soldiers were on the beach, ready to intercept the vessel as it came to shore.

The soldiers detained the four men on board, and hidden beneath the seats were 2,000 pounds of cocaine, worth an estimated $14 million.

It was the biggest drug bust ever recorded by the NORFORCE Unit, and I was there to see it with my own eyes.

But of course, I didn't care about the drugs.

All I cared about was how Bunji had seen the vessel from so far away, when not a single US marine could – even though all of us had 20/20 vision ourselves.

And that's when I got the breakthrough I'd been praying for.

After quizzing Bunji about it, I discovered to my amazement that the eyesight of Aboriginal people in outback Australia is up to FOUR TIMES better than ours.

This ability has become known as 'super sight.'

I've since discovered that the vision of Australian Aboriginals is the best in the world. Professor Hugh Taylor from the University of Melbourne's Indigenous Health unit commented on Prince Harry's training with the NORFORCE unit in 2015...

He may need to get a pair of binoculars to see what they see with their naked eye (22).

Scientists consider good vision to be 6:6 vision. That means that a person standing 20 feet away from an eye chart can see it as clearly as an average person standing 20 feet away.

But, for the Aboriginal people, general vision is much better.

Professor Taylor stated that

*The vision of the Aboriginal people, the fineness of their vision, **is better than has been reported anywhere else in the world.***

Professor Taylor's research backs this up. Studies have shown that some Aboriginal people in the Northern Territory, Western Australia and South Australia had **6:1.4 vision**. This means that they could see things from 20 feet away that an average person could only see from 4.5 feet way.

Professor Taylor provides a historical example of how finely tuned the vision of the Aboriginal people were. Astronomers were looking back at records from the 1840s into Aboriginal descriptions of constellations.

The astronomers were unable to figure out how the constellations worked. After discussing the situation with Professor Taylor, they went back with binoculars. Then, they were able to pick out all of the missing stars that the Aboriginal people could see with the naked eye (23).

The question now racing through my mind was, Why?

Why are the Aboriginal people blessed with such superior eyesight?

Was it genetic, environmental or something else?

That's why I cornered Bunji one night. I told him all about my wife's condition, stressing that she didn't have long to go until she lost her sight completely.

'If you know anything that can help her, please tell me,' I pleaded.

Bunji smiled, patted me on the shoulder, and told me to wait where I was.

A few minutes later, he returned with a notepad and pencil, and began to scribble down what looked like a recipe, complete with a list of strange foods, most of which I'd never even heard of.

'What's this?' I asked him, looking down the list.

'The secret you've been searching for,' he said, with a glint in his eye.

'Our super sight is all down to the land we live on,' he continued, mysteriously.

'This recipe has been in my family for generations,' he said. 'Eat these foods and your wife will recover.'

With that, Bunji stood up, gave me a knowing smile, and rejoined his unit. I never saw him again.

But I had his list – and just maybe that would be all I needed.

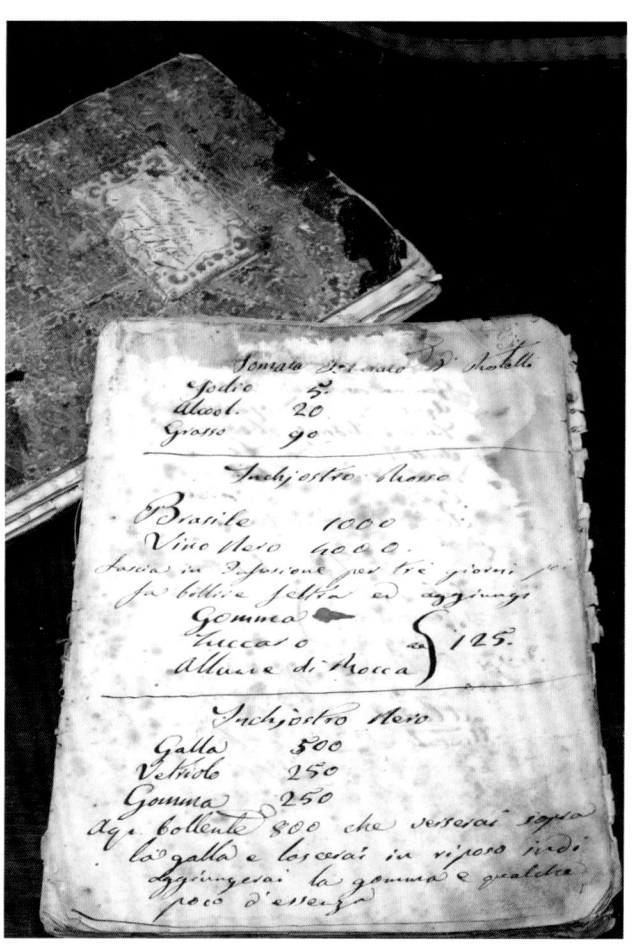

The moment I returned to the United States, I threw myself into researching the ingredients that he had jotted down that night.

What I found was shocking.

There were trials upon trials, including The Age-Related Eye Disease Study, or AREDS, the gold standard study into vision loss carried out by the National Eye Institute, which proved beyond any doubt that the ingredients Bunji had jotted down contained specific compounds that are absolutely ESSENTIAL to vision (24).

The two key nutrients, lutein and zeaxanthin, are *the* two most important nutrients to eat, because they're EXACTLY what our eyes need to ward off vision problems like macular degeneration, cataracts, glaucoma, and even near and farsightedness.

The AREDS study found that people diagnosed with early AMD who ate these two nutrients were 25-30% less likely to go on to develop advanced AMD, while they also reduced their risk of developing central vision loss by 19%.

Another study of the elderly Finnish population published in the *British Journal of Nutrition* reported that 'high plasma concentrations of lutein and zeaxanthin reduced the risk of age-related cataracts by a massive 41%' (25).

That's great news, considering that age-related cataracts are one of the leading causes of visual impairment in the United States, with the number of Americans likely to be affected set to increase to an estimated 30 million by 2020.

In the next chapter, we focus on these two vital nutrients that have the power to transform your vision.

Bunji's List

So, what are the magic foods that Bunji listed for me on that life-changing night in the Outback?

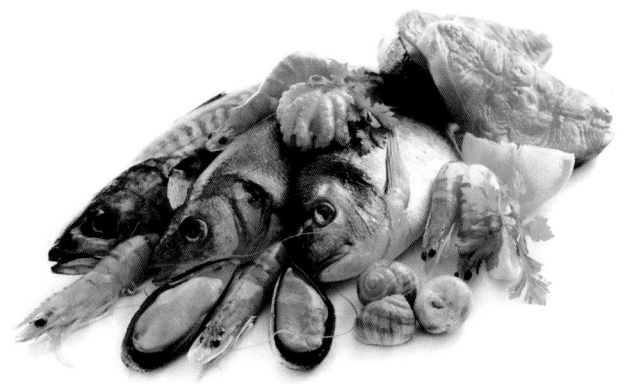

In this section, we consider each of them. These are the very foods that the Aboriginal people of Australia have been consuming for thousands of years – and that have given them the best eyesight of any people on the planet! (Note: Many of these foods aren't readily available to many people, especially in the United States.)

Fish and Shellfish

For thousands of years, the Aboriginal people have relied on the sea as a primary food source. The food type was dependent on the season and the part of the country. Creeks, rivers, beaches, islands, and coastal and sea areas were all rich food sources. From them, the following were taken...

- Baramundi
- Jewfish
- Catfish
- Cod
- Eels
- Grunter
- Prawns
- Crayfish
- Oysters
- Periwinkle
- Stingray

- Shark
- Crabs
- Turtles
- Turtle eggs
- Dugongs
- Clam
- Triton

What My Research Uncovered...

A recent study found that seniors who ate at least one serving of fish per week were 60% less likely to suffer from macular degeneration. Seafoods are rich in zinc, which help to ward off macular degeneration.

Seafoods are also rich in Omega-3 fatty acids, which are essential for eye health. The study just mentioned also showed that seniors who ate shellfish on a weekly basis were far less likely to develop macular degeneration. Researchers asked 2,391 people between the ages of 65 and 84 how much fish and shellfish they ate. Those who consumed the most fish had by far the best eyesight (26) (27).

Two Omega-3 fatty acids that are especially important for eye health are

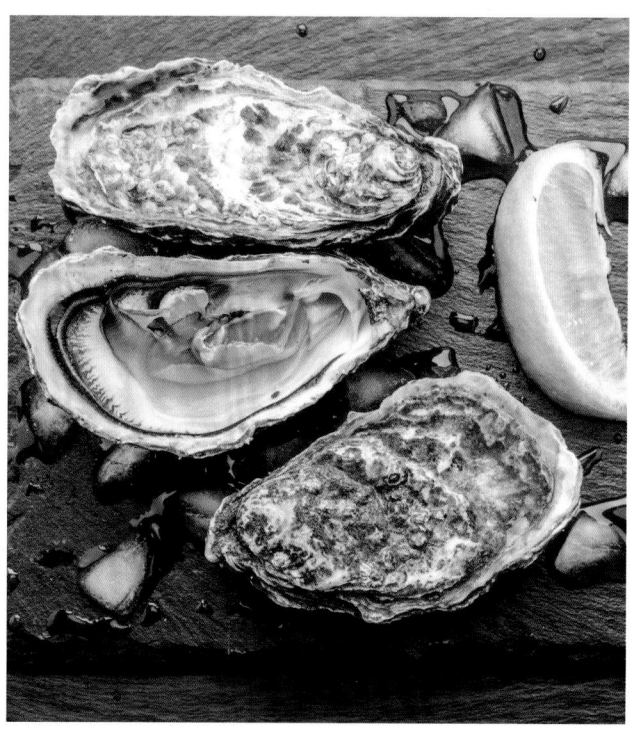

Docosahexaenoic Acid (DHA) and Eicosapentaenoic Acid (EPA). The highest concentrations of DHA in the body is in the retina. EPA is necessary to make DHA. If you don't get enough of both of these fatty acids, you will likely develop dry eye syndrome (28) (29) (30).

A 2005 study involving more than 40,000 women showed that participants who ate less than the minimum recommended amount of these good fats had a greatly increased risk of developing dry eye syndrome. All types of fish are excellent sources of DHA and EPA (31) (32) (33) (34).

Animal Organ Meats

Animal organ meats are the organs of animals that we prepare as food. They are also known as offal. In the Western world, we overwhelmingly rely on muscle meats and tend to discard the organs. However, the Aboriginals have been consuming organ meats for centuries. These include the heart, liver, brains, intestines and even the testicles of the emu, kangaroo, koala, platypus, Tasmanian Devil, and a large variety of snakes.

Organ meats are extremely nutritious if they come from toxin-free, grass-fed, free-range animals that were not exposed to chemical fertilizers and pesticides. They are, in fact, more nutrient dense than muscle meat. They are especially high in the B-vitamins B12 and folate. Many studies have shown that B12 is essential for eye health. A 100gram serving of cooked beef liver provides you with a staggering 1,386% of the RDI (35).

Green and Kakadu Plum

Green plums are tart, crunchy plums that don't have much taste, neither bitter nor sour. But they sure pack a lot of nutritional power. Green plums are excellent sources of Vitamins A, C and K. They are also heart healthy, rich in antioxidants and full of fiber. Green plums are low in calories. They also support the body's absorption of calcium.

Green plums are rich in both lutein and zeaxanthin, which, as we've seen, are the two most important nutrients for eye health. Vitamin A allows the eyes to absorb light by keeping the membranes in the eyes strong. It also reduces the risk of night blindness.

The kakadu plum grows across the top end of the northern part of Australia. It has been identified as the world's richest source of Vitamin C. There are 3,000 mg of Vitamin C in every 100

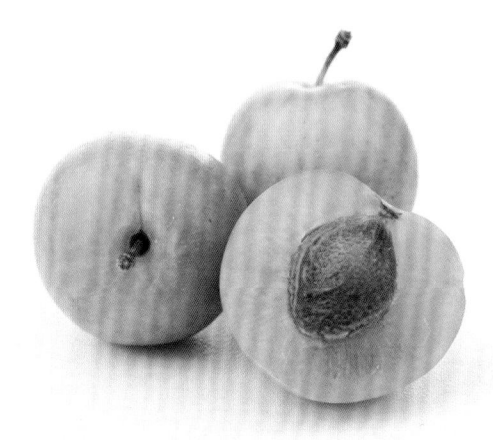

grams of kakadu plum. That is 50 times more Vitamin C than you will get out of an orange! (36)

The kakadu plum contains a couple of very important phytochemicals:

- Gallic Acid
- Ellagic Acid

Gallic acid has potent antibacterial, antiviral and antifungal properties. It is also a powerful anti-inflammatory, which makes it great for fighting the free radical damage that leads to deteriorating eyesight.

Ellagic acid has anticarcinogenic effects against a wide range of carcinogens in human tissue.

Wild / Bush Tomatoes

The bush tomato is the fruit of a small desert plant. Of the more than 100 species of wild tomatoes that grow in Australia, only six of them are edible. They are very high in Vitamin C and potassium.

As well as eating the fruit of the bush tomato plant, the Aboriginals also eat

the roots of the plant. The roots were baked in ash and then peeled back and placed in the mouth to treat toothache (37).

Quandong

Quandong is a type of wild peach that grows on a small desert tree that reaches up to 13 feet in height. The Quandong tree is unique in that it uses the root system of other trees, as well as shrubs and grasses, to supplement its water and nutrient supply. For that reason, it is often found growing at the base of other trees.

The fruit of this tree is a bright scarlet color. It is less than an inch in diameter. Inside is a large nut or kernel. The taste is a little tart. This fruit has more than twice the amount of Vitamin C as an orange. The kernel is also very nutritious (38).

Pigweed

The pigweed plant is a succulent ground creeper that produces small fruits or seeds. Aboriginals grind the seeds into a paste. The leaves and shoots of the pigweed plant are eaten raw.

The seeds of the pigweed are oily and highly nutritious. They are high in fiber, protein and magnesium, as well as iron. The leaves of the pigweed plant are also very high in Vitamins A and C, both of which are vital for eye health. Taking a cupful of pigweed leaves daily would provide you with 73% of the RDA for Vitamin C and 90% of the RDA for Vitamin A. This plant is also very high in manganese, calcium and magnesium, phosphorous, potassium, zinc and copper.

Pigweed leaves are a great source of Omega-3 fatty acids, providing 1.3 mg per cupful with only a tenth of a gram of fat (39).

Wattleseed

Wattleseed is the flower of the acacia tree. There are a huge range of types of acacia that grow across of Australia. The seed of the Acacia tree is very hardy. Upon falling to the ground, it can last for up to 20 years. The hardy outer casing protects the seed inside. The seed has been a rich source of protein and carbohydrates for the Aboriginal people for centuries.

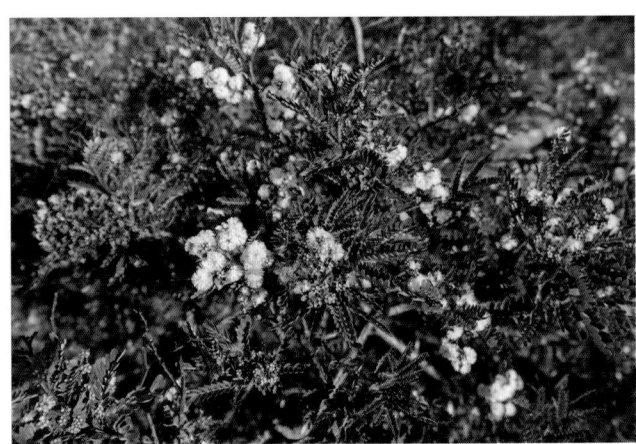

Aboriginal people would grind the wattleseed into a flour between flat grinding stones. They would then cook it into cakes or damper. It has a nutty, mild coffee flavor.

These seeds are a rich source of potassium, calcium, iron and zinc. They also contain more than 30% of their content in fiber (40).

Witchetty Grubs

The Witchetty Grub is the larvae of a moth that is only found in central Australia. They live in the roots of the witchetty bush and the Bloodwood tree. The grub tastes like scrambled eggs. The most commonly eaten type of witchetty grub is the larvae of the Cossid Moth.

The witchetty grub is very high in protein. It is also rich in Vitamin C. In fact, six witchetty grubs provide as much Vitamin C as an orange. They are also rich in Vitamin B1, which boosts energy and helps maintain the nervous system.

Crushing witchetty grubs and placing them on burns also helps the skin heal (41).

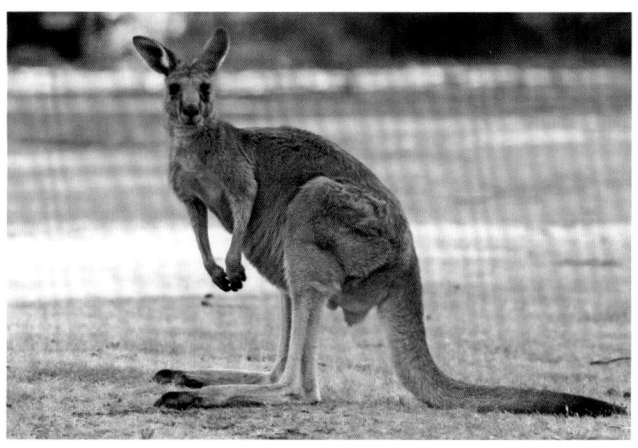

Kangaroo Meat

Kangaroo is a very healthy red meat source. It is very lean, high in protein and rich in essential minerals, such as iron and zinc. A 200gram serving of grilled kangaroo steak provides you with a huge 42 grams of protein, with only 2.6 grams of fat. Better still, you get all of this in just 196 calories.

Kangaroo meat also contains the essential Omega-3 fatty acids DHA and EPA. The fat in kangaroo meat is also healthy for humans. Forty percent of kangaroo meat consists of long chain polyunsaturated fatty acids (PUFAs). These improve blood flow, reduce the blood's clotting tendency and reduce the risk of heart attack and stroke.

A study conducted by Professor Kerin O'Dea, Director of the Menzies School of Health Research in Darwin, Australia showed that Aborigines who returned to a traditional, kangaroo meat rich diet displayed dramatic improvements in diabetes and other risk factors for cardiovascular diseases. They also had marked improvements in eyesight (42).

Emu Meat

The red meat of the Emu has been consumed by Aboriginals for thousands of years. It is very low in fat and cholesterol, but high in protein. This makes it very lean (97% fat-free). It contains more Vitamin A, Vitamin C and Vitamin B12 than chicken. All three of these vitamins are essential for eye health (43).

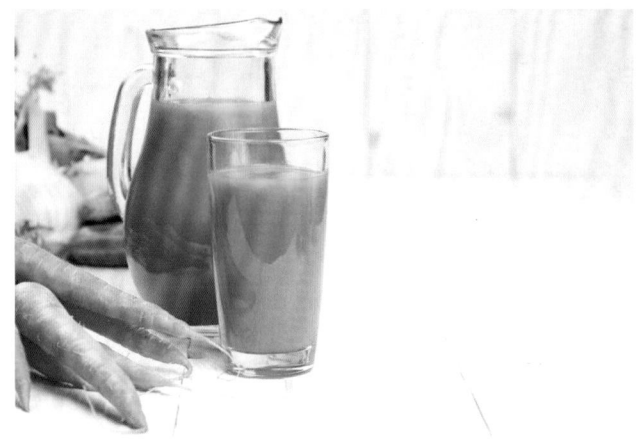

Carrots

Of all the foods we could eat for improved eyesight, carrots are by far the most well known. From the time we could walk, our parents told us to eat our carrots for good eyesight. It turns out that mom and dad knew what they were talking about.

Aboriginals were keen consumers of wild carrots. Here's why they are so good for your vision…

- Carrots are rich in beta-carotene. Beta-carotene is a precursor for Vitamin D. Vitamin D deficiency is the leading cause of blindness in the developing world.
- Carrots are high in Vitamin A, which is essential for preventing cataracts and macular degeneration. It also wards off Xerophthalmia, which is a disease characterized by dry eyes, swollen eyelids and corneal ulcers.
- Carrots are rich in lutein, which increases the density of pigments in the macula (44).

Finger Lime

The finger lime is a delicate rainforest tree that is grown in southeastern Queensland and Victoria in Australia. The fruit is green and cylindrical in shape, about four inches long and about an inch in diameter. They have large thorns and contain seeds. The fruit contains an acidic juice that is similar to a lime.

The finger lime is very high in Vitamin C, as well as antioxidants, B Vitamins and potassium. Eating finger limes is believed to reduce the risk of mouth, stomach and throat cancer by 50%. It is also very high in antioxidants, which helps lower the risk of cardiovascular disease and macular degeneration. Finger limes also contain polyphenols and beta carotene for a healthy immune system.

Finger limes are a rich source of both lutein and zeaxanthins (45).

Kutjera

The kutjera is a bush food plant that grows in arid regions of Australia. It grows on a small shrub with green leaves. It produces purple flowers and an edible small fruit, which is yellow when ripe and then becomes brown. It looks much like a raisin.

The fruit of the kutjera is rich in Vitamin C. The taste is similar to tamarillo and caramel (46).

Muntries

Muntries are also known as emu apples. They are a low-growing plant found along the southern coast of Australia. The plant produces a fruit that is about a half inch in diameter. At maturity, they are green with a tinge of red. They taste like a spicy apple.

Muntries are extremely rich in antioxidants, containing more than blueberries. They also contain natural oils and waxes that are great for replenishing the skin (47).

Riberry

The Riberry is a small red fruit found along the Australian east coast. Aboriginals referred to them as the 'medicine berry.' They are rich in essential vitamins and minerals that keep the immune system healthy and strong.

The riberry fruit contains three times as much folate as blueberries. It is also rich in manganese and calcium, and contains high levels of anthocyanin, which is a potent antioxidant that improves cognitive functioning and vision (48).

Davidson's Plum

Davidson's Plum is grown in four varieties from Australia's tropical north to New South Wales. The fruit is between one and two and a half inches in diameter. It has a blood-red flesh and either one or two seeds. It has more than 100 times the Vitamin C you would get from an orange. It is also rich in lutein, along with magnesium, zinc, calcium, potassium and manganese (49).

CHAPTER **NINE**

THE TWO SUPER NUTRIENTS THAT CAN RESTORE YOUR EYESIGHT

My Outback Adventure, during which I met Bunji, was the catalyst that led to my discovery of the two most amazing super nutrients that exist when it comes to improving and protecting your vision. The list of foods that Bunji had scribbled on a piece of paper and handed to me when I'd pleaded with him for help with my wife's rapidly deteriorating eyesight were abundant in these two nutrients. They are:

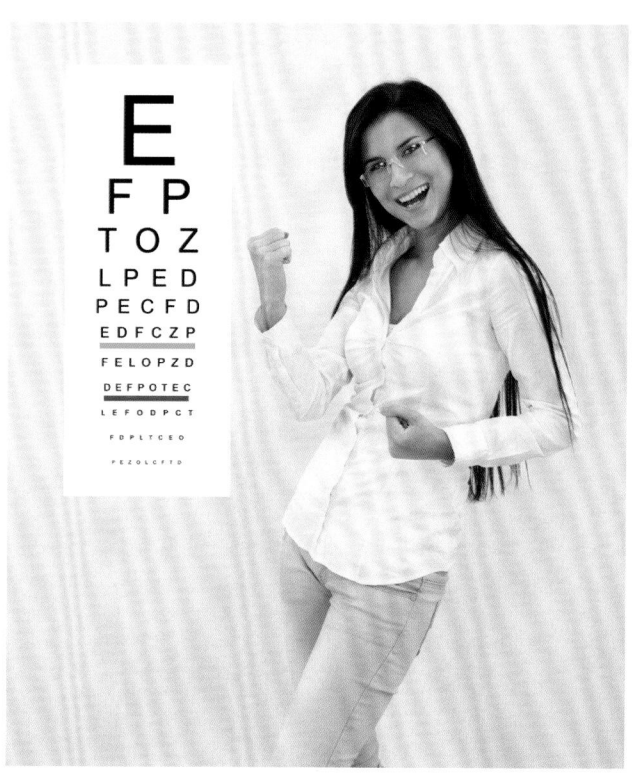

- Lutein
- Zeaxanthin

Let's learn more about them.

Lutein and zeaxanthin are carotenoids. Carotenoids are the plant pigments that give color to many fruits and vegetables. These particular two carotenoids are deposited in the eyes. Of the more than 600 carotenoids that we get from nature, only about 20 of them accumulate in the eyes. And of those 20, only lutein and zeaxanthin build up in the macular region of the eye.

Lutein and zeaxanthin have powerful antioxidant properties. That makes them the ideal defense against free radical damage to the macular region. This free radical damage is caused by such factors as bad diet, overexposure to the sun, and ultraviolet light.

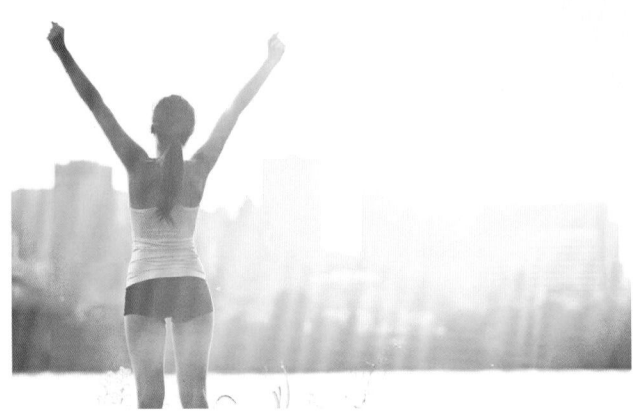

Of course, we need sunlight in order to see. But some of the ultraviolet light that goes through the pupil to the retina at the back of the eye can actually generate free radicals, causing damage to the optic nerves and the tissue around them. This can slowly lead to macular degeneration and, if unchecked, blindness.

Because lutein and zeaxanthin concentrate in the area of the eye known as the macula lutea, they act as an antioxidant. They actually have the ability to absorb the ultraviolet light, decreasing free radical damage to the eye. They quash the free radicals before they can do extensive damage.

So, we need to have a certain amount of lutein in the eye in order to prevent eye damage from occurring over our lifetimes. But, it has also been shown to dramatically improve existing eye problems (50).

One study, published in the journal *Optometry* in 2007, looked at the effect of giving lutein supplementation to 13 patients with retinitis pigmentosa and three patients with macular degeneration. Both groups had significant improvement in their vision when given 40 mg of lutein daily for the first nine weeks, with a reduction to 20mg per day for the next 17 weeks (51).

In another study, two individuals who consumed 30 mg of lutein per day demonstrated an improvement in macular pigment optical density by 39% in one subject and 21% in the other. This improvement in the optical density of the macular pigment reduced the amount of harmful ultraviolet light reaching the photoreceptors by 30 to 40% (52).

Studies Involving Cataracts

Cataracts have caused between 30 and 50 million people worldwide to lose their eyesight. This condition results in opacification of the lens of the eye. This obstructs the passage of

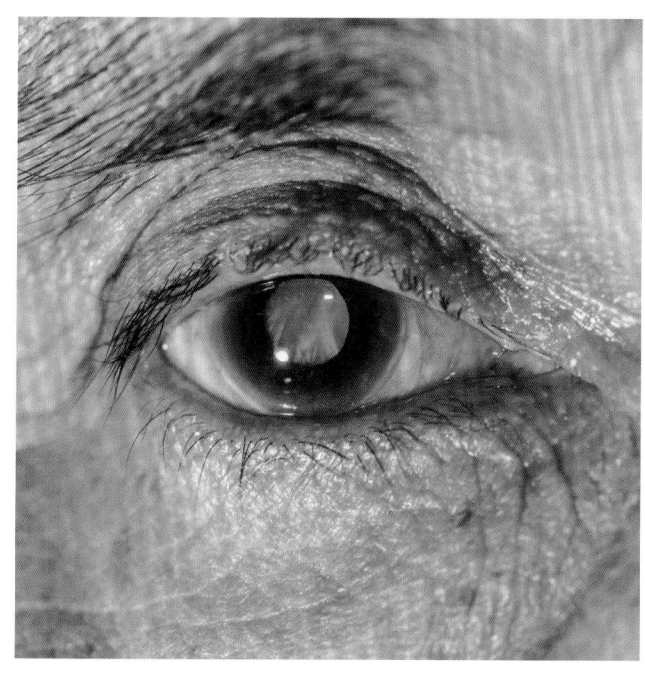

light, resulting in impaired vision and potential blindness (53).

Cataracts become more common with increasing age, and is a leading cause of disability among the elderly population throughout the world. More than one million cataract extractions are performed annually in the US.

Researchers have long believed that lutein and zeaxanthin play a crucial role in the prevention of the oxidation of lens proteins and the formation of cataracts (57).

Epidemiological studies examining the relation of dietary intake and blood levels of lutein plus zeaxanthin with

the risk of cataract show that these two compounds have a hugely beneficial effect (58).

One Spanish study investigated the effect of lutein on cataracts. Over a period of two years, lutein and Vitamin E antioxidant supplementation was given to 17 people with cataracts. Supplementation with both nutrients improved cataracts, but the greatest improvement was seen with lutein. In the double-blind study, participants took 15 mg of lutein and 100 mg of Vitamin E or a placebo three times per week for up to two years. The researchers regularly measured serum carotenoid levels. Visual performance was also monitored. A significant improvement in visual acuity and glare sensitivity was seen in the lutein group only (54).

In the Beaver Dam Eye Study (BDES), patients with cataracts aged 43 to 84 years were studied with a range of antioxidants. Lutein was the only examined carotenoid associated with significant cataract improvement (59).

Likewise, the results of the Nurse Health Study (NHS) and the US Health Professionals Follow-up Study (HPFS) showed that subjects with the highest intake of lutein and zeaxanthin had a 22% or 19% decreased risk of cataract extraction regardless of gender (60) (61).

Increasing intake of foods rich in lutein, such as spinach and kale, was most consistently associated with a lower risk of cataracts, while cataracts were not strongly associated with consumption of carotene-rich foods (62) (63) (64) (65).

Where Do We Get Lutein and Zeaxanthin?

The human body is unable to make its own lutein and zeaxanthin. As a result, we depend entirely on dietary sources for these essential eye compounds. Lutein is present in a wide variety of plant foods, especially in dark green leafy vegetables. The two foods that have the highest amount are **spinach** and **kale**.

Other major sources include broccoli, turnip greens, summer squash, and Brussels sprouts. Dietary sources of zeaxanthin are limited to green, certain yellow–orange fruits and vegetables, most abundantly in **nectarine**, **orange** and **papaya**.

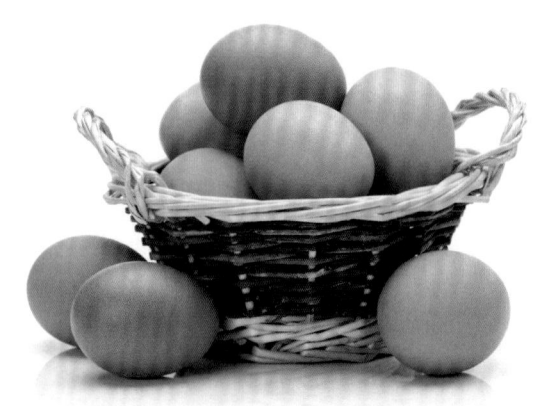

Eggs, though not the richest dietary source of lutein and zeaxanthin, are considered a good source of these carotenoids due to the high bioavailability of lutein and zeaxanthin from the lipid matrix of the yolks.

The Top 10 Sources of Lutein and Zeaxanthin

Kale (1 cup = 22mg)

Turnip Greens (1/2 cup = 9 mg)

Collard Greens (1/2 cup = 8.7 mg)

Spinach (1 cup = 6.7 mg)

Broccoli (1 cup = 3.3 mg)

Brussels Sprouts (1 cup = 2 mg)

Corn (1 cup = 1.4 mg) [In moderation.]

Green Beans (1 cup = 0.8 mg) [In moderation.]

Eggs (2 whole = 0.3 mg)

Orange (1 medium = 0.2 mg)

How Much Lutein Do We Need?

There is no general recommendation for the daily intake of lutein and zeaxanthin. The general consensus among experts, however, is to have a minimum of **10 mg** of lutein and the same amount of zeaxanthin per day (65).

Getting 10 mg minimum per day is not difficult. As you can see in the list above, a cup of kale will provide you with 22 grams.

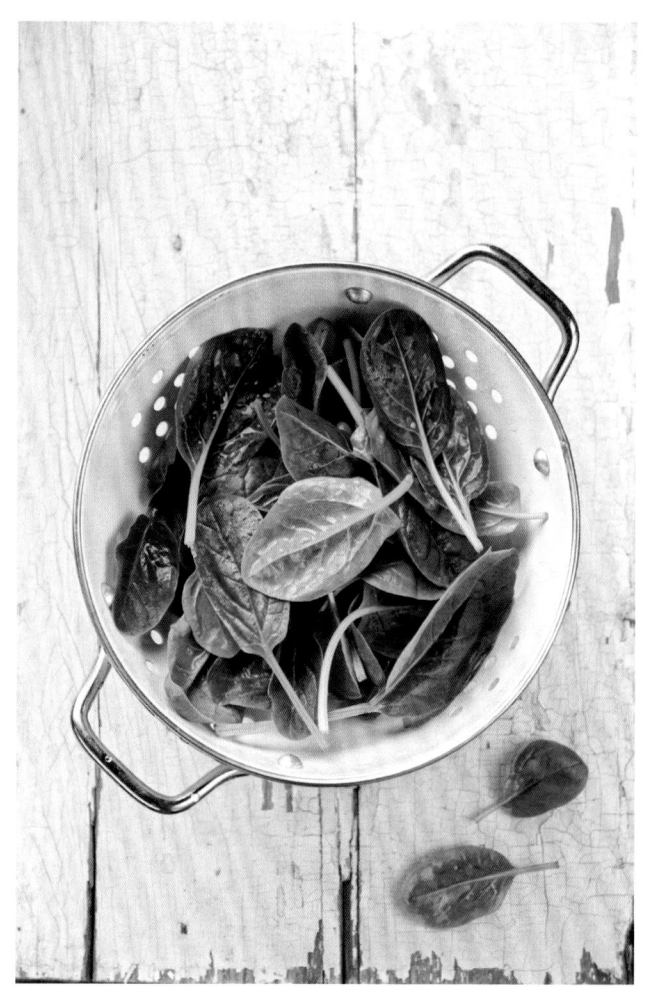

Each of the recipes in our 21-day protocol will guarantee that you exceed 10 mg of these vital, vision-enhancing nutrients every day.

CHAPTER **TEN**

THE ESSENTIAL EIGHT ANTIOXIDANTS FOR EYESIGHT

The list of essential foods that Bunji handed to me in the Australian outback contained lutein and zeaxanthin in abundance. But, as I began researching those foods, I discovered that there were other nutrients that kept cropping up as well. Eventually, I managed to formulate a list of eight essential antioxidants.

My next step was to see what the scientific literature had to say about these nutrients. Would Western medicine back up the wisdom of Aboriginals?

What I discovered floored me.

Every single one of the foods that Bunji had put on his list was packed with nutrients that the Western scientific community was only now discovering to be ultra-effective vision enhancers.

Here's the list:

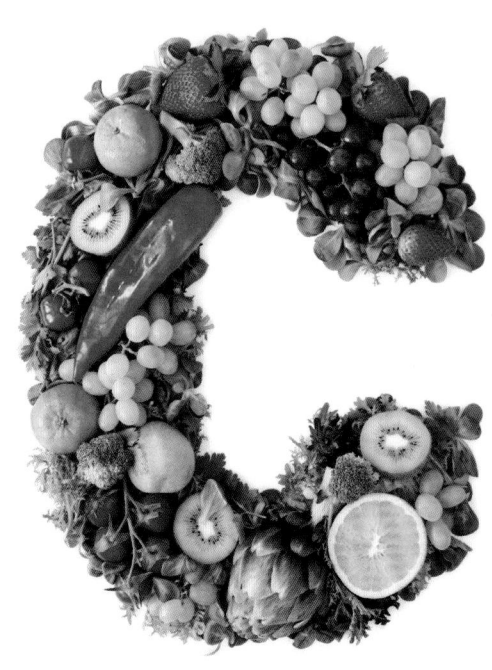

- Lutein
- Zeaxanthin
- Omega-3
- Vitamin B6
- Vitamin B12
- Vitamin A
- Vitamin C
- Zinc

You already know about the first two. In this chapter, we take a closer look at the remaining six, one at a time.

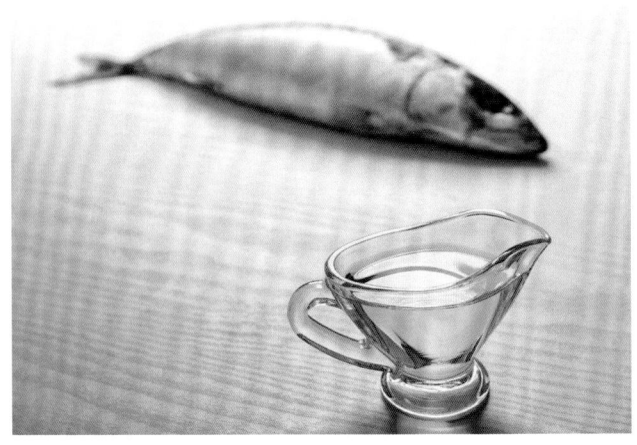

Essential Nutrient #1: Omega-3 Fatty Acids

The majority of unsaturated fats are liquid at room temperature and mainly come from plant sources. They come under two subcategories:

- Monounsaturated fats
- Polyunsaturated fats

Polyunsaturated fats are unique because they contain Essential Fatty Acids (EFAs). EFAs are the fatty acids that your body cannot produce and that must be provided through the diet. The two main EFAs are

✓ Omega-3
✓ Omega-6

The modern Western diet provides these two essential fats at the startling ratio of **20:1 in favor of Omega-6**. That means that most people are chronically short of Omega-3 fatty acids.

The reason?

Omega-6 is contained in refined grains as well as in animals fed grains. The emphasis on wheat products and animal meats that has characterized our eating pattern over the last hundred years has done a good job of giving us our Omega-6, but an absolutely lousy job when it comes to Omega-3.

This imbalance has, of itself, caused some major problems. It has caused us to be far more prone to inflammatory and cardiovascular diseases that never used to affect humans.

Getting more Omega-3 fatty acids into your body will revolutionize the way your body looks, feels and acts, especially in relation to your vision. The highest concentration of Omega-3 DHA fatty acids is in the delicate photoreceptors of your eye. As Omega-3 levels get lower and lower in the body, the eyes are the first to go.

Good sources of Omega-3:
- **Walnuts**
- **Seeds**
- **Fish oil**
- **Krill oil**
- **Flaxseed oil**

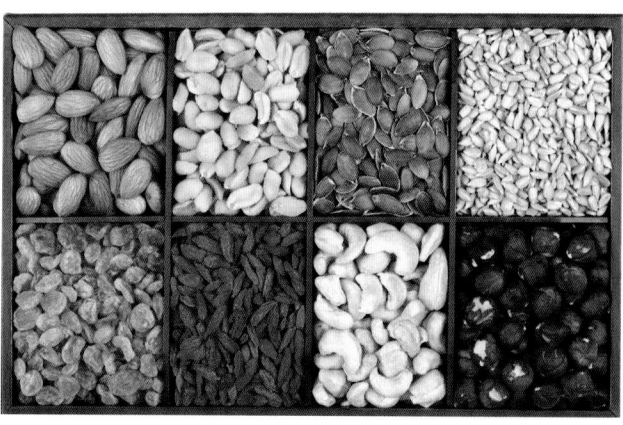

Omega-3 and Dry Eye

The tear film that coats the front of the eye is very complex. Its outer layer is an oily, thin layer produced by special glands called Meibomian glands. The lipid layer serves to lubricate and prevent evaporation of the saltwater middle layer. The middle watery layer nourishes and protects the cornea. The inner layer is a native mucous that is secreted from cells in the front surface of the eye. It is important in helping the middle layer spread evenly across to the front of the eye.

Blinking causes excess tears to be pushed out of a drainage system that leads from the inner corner of the eyelids to the nose. Anything that causes interruption of blinking, such as staring at a computer, wind or blowing fans, can compromise your tears.

A dry eye surface can also result from medications like oral antihistamines and antidepressants. Medical conditions including arthritis and menopause, with fluctuating hormones, can also cause dry eye. In some cases, poor tear quality and reduced tear quantity have no specific causes and are simply due to the aging process.

Dry eye can range from a mild, dry surface to a very disrupted tear film. The main symptoms of dry eye are

- Watery eyes or excess tearing
- Burning
- Gritty
- 'Sand in the eyes'
- Itching
- Discomfort
- Red eyes
- Blurry vision

People suffering from dry eye might actually experience excessive tearing while the tear gland tries to relieve the dry eye condition itself. It may produce low quality, unwanted tears in order to coat the eye. When tear levels are low, the eye senses burning, itching and discomfort. If the condition worsens, the eyes can become red and vision can become blurry. The tears that are released to combat these issues leave you with nothing but watery eyes.

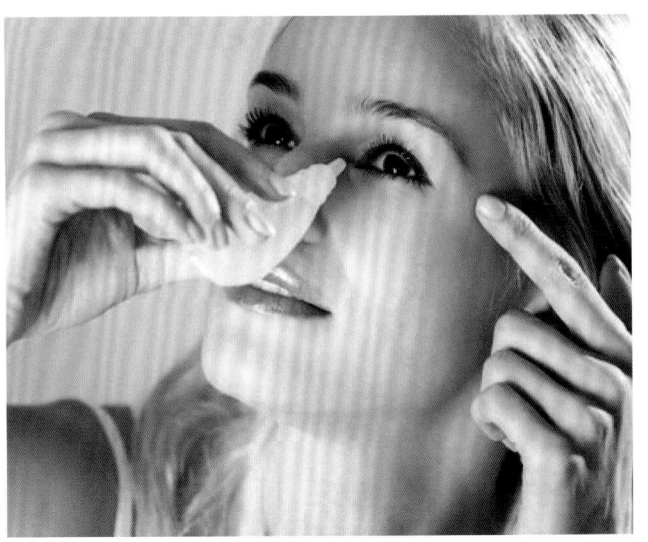

Treatment of dry eye is necessary to restore a healthy ocular surface. Treatments range from warm compresses to simple artificial tears and ointments. However, these treatments fail to address the underlying cause of dry eye...

Meibomian Gland Dysfunction (MGD)

There are approximately 31 Meibomian glands in the upper eyelid, with 26 in the lower eyelid. The glands in the upper eyelid are longer and produce more oil. Each gland contains little pockets that act like an oil factory, producing oil and pushing it out into the duct to exit the eyelid.

The muscle inside your eyelid assists in milking the glands, pushing the oil into the opening and out onto the eye. Upon exiting the duct and being pushed onto your eye, the oil then forms the outer layer of tears, called the lipid layer. This oily outer layer serves to prevent evaporation of the watery middle layer. The layer that sits against the eyeball is made of mucous secreted from cells in the front surface of the eye. It is important in helping the outer layer spread evenly across the surface of the eye.

MGD is a chronic dysfunction of the Meibomian glands. This is normally characterized by severe duct obstruction; this results in lowered oil secretion, which leads to a decrease in the quality of the tear film eye irritation and possible ocular disease.

MGD is chronic, which means that it is long term. Medical science does not have a cure for this condition. All we can do is treat the symptoms. Symptom relief will occur when treatment is actively occurring, but symptoms will return if treatment stops.

Effective treatment for dry eye involves unblocking the exit to the Meibomian gland. When this exit is blocked, you are also more prone to styes, as well as to bumps on the eyelid. The reason for this is that the gland keeps producing oil that has nowhere to go, thereby forming a lump.

The oil that is being produced when you have MGD is not high quality oil. Treatment should involve both unblocking the channel to allow oil to the eye and improving the quality of the oil.

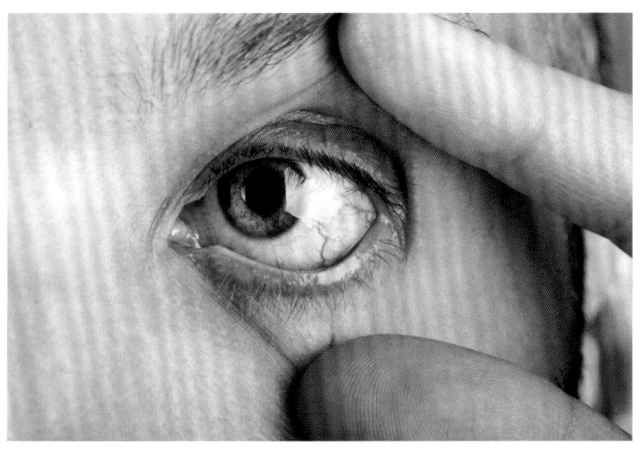

Diet plays a critical role in the oil production of the Meibomian gland.

A diet that is high in Omega-6 fatty acids – the typical Western diet – will produce lower-quality oils and will increase inflammation.

Both of these will result in increased dryness and eye inflammation. As discussed, Americans obtain an excessive amount of Omeg-6 fatty acids through their consumption of beef, dairy, vegetable shortening and cooking oils. Such foods as hamburgers, cheeseburgers, pizza and potato chips all contain high amounts of Omega-6 fatty acids.

While the ratio of Omega-6 to Omega-3 should be 1:4, it is much closer to 1:20 for most people in developed countries.

Omega-3 fatty acids are especially beneficial in treating dry eye syndrome. Taking in more Omega-3 rich foods will dramatically improve the health of your eyes, as well as your skin, hair and fingernails. Omega-3 fatty acids ***decrease inflammation of the eye and help the glands to produce better quality oil***. This leads to fewer dryness symptoms and more comfort throughout the day.

There have also been studies that have shown a link between increased intake of Omega-3 fatty acids and defense against macular degeneration.

One series of studies, which was published in the journal *Pediatrics* and carried out by researchers at Harvard Medical School, showed that healthy preterm babies who were given an Omega-3 supplement displayed markedly better visual acuity at 2 - 4 months of age when compared with preterm babies who were not given Omega-3.

A Canadian study that was published in the *American Journal of Clinical Nutrition* showed that the children of pregnant women who supplemented with Omega-3 from the fourth month of pregnancy onward were far more likely to have improved visual acuity at two months of age than babies whose mothers did not supplement with Omega-3 (66).

A large-scale 2008 study showed that an adult study group who ate oily fish once per week had half the risk of developing macular degeneration when compared to a control group (67).

In a 2009 National Eyes Institute study, information was used from the AREDS study to examine the effect of Omega-3 on eye health. It was found that patients who had the highest levels of Omega-3 in their diet were 30% less likely to develop macular degeneration over a 12-year period than those who consumed small amounts of Omega-3 (68).

AREDS 2, the 2013 follow up to the original AREDS study, confirmed that daily supplementation with Omega-3 fatty acids, when combined with the original nutrient recommendations of beta-carotene, Vitamin-C, Vitamin-E, zinc and copper, would decrease the risk of age-related macular degeneration (69).

Finally, a study of more than 32,000 women, aged between 45 and 64, revealed that the women who had the highest Omega-6 to Omega-3 ratio (15:1), had a much greater risk of getting dry eye syndrome compared with women with a ratio of 4:1 (70).

Essential Nutrient #2: Vitamin B6

Vitamin B6 is also known as pyridoxine, or the mood vitamin. It helps cognitive and other brain functions by increasing serotonin levels and protects the nerves that send signals back and forth. Recent studies have also shown that it can play an important role in preventing macular degeneration.

B6 is made up of three related compounds, namely pyridoxine, pyridoxamine and pyridoxal. This coenzyme is essential for protein metabolism. It is necessary for the release of energy in forms that the cells can use. It is also important in the functioning of the nervous and immune systems, as well as the manufacture of red blood cells. B6 also helps the body manufacture hemoglobin, the carrier of oxygen in the blood. It assists in maintaining blood sugar homeostasis as well.

B6 has proven to be an important heart disease preventative. We rely on this vitamin every day, as it is needed for movement, memory, energy expenditure and blood flow. A deficiency in Vitamin B6 can, therefore, lead to a whole range of different symptoms, including impaired vision.

Studies on the specific effects of Vitamin B6 on vision are limited. Those that have been conducted, however, are very encouraging.

One large study showed that women who took 50 mg of Vitamin B6 every day, in conjunction with 1,000 mg of Vitamin B12 and 2,500 mg of folic acid, were able to significantly reduce their risk of developing age-related macular degeneration (AMD) (71).

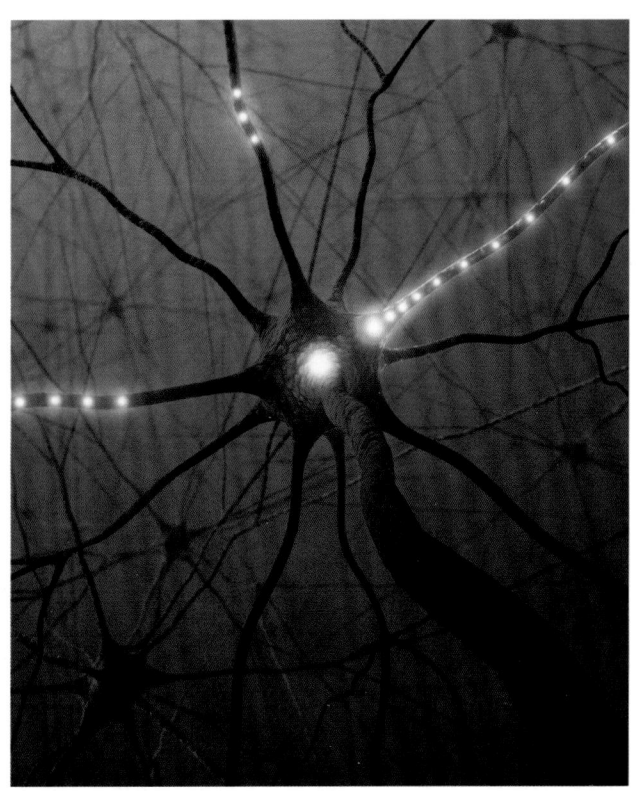

How does Vitamin B6 help prevent macular degeneration?

It does so by helping us absorb magnesium, which is used in the production of tears. This helps to keep the eyes lubricated, healthy and clear.

Where Do We Source Vitamin B6?

As with the other B vitamins, Vitamin B6 is water soluble. That means that it cannot be stored by the body and must be obtained through the foods we eat.

The following foods are highest in Vitamin B6:

Dried Herbs and Spices

Although dried herbs and spices are rarely used in large portions, adding in a few extra pinches to your sauces, soups and stews is a great way to get more vitamin B6 into your diet. Chili powder contains the most Vitamin B6, with 3.67 mg per 100 g serving (184% of the RDA) or 0.294 mg (15% of the RDA) per tablespoon. Chili powder is followed by paprika, which has 0.28 mg (14% of the RDA) per tablespoon,

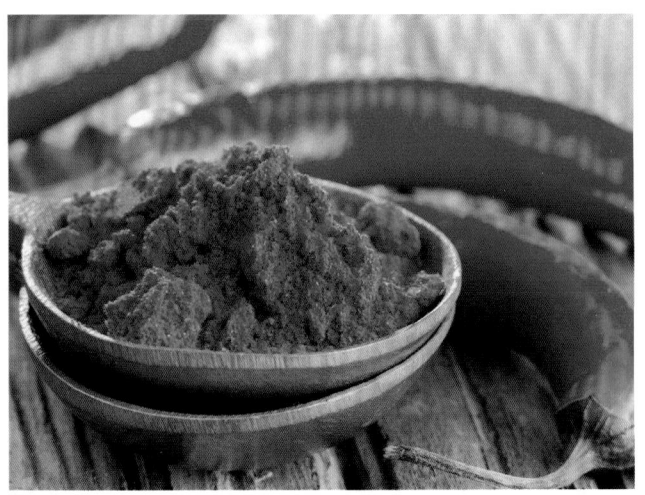

garlic powder (12% of the RDA per tablespoon), dried tarragon (6% of the RDA), ground sage (3% of the RDA), dried spearmint (3% of the RDA), basil, chives, savory, turmeric, bay leaves, rosemary, dill, onion powder, oregano and marjoram.

Pistachios

Pistachios are a delicious snack and a great addition to salads. One hundred grams of raw pistachios (~3/4 cup) will provide 1.7 mg (85% RDA) of vitamin B6. That is 0.48 mg (24% RDA) per ounce (~49 pistachios). Try to eat raw pistachios, instead of roasted pistachios which contain considerably less vitamin B6. Roasted pistachios will provide 1.27 mg (64% RDA) per 100gram serving, or 0.36 mg (18% RDA) per ounce.

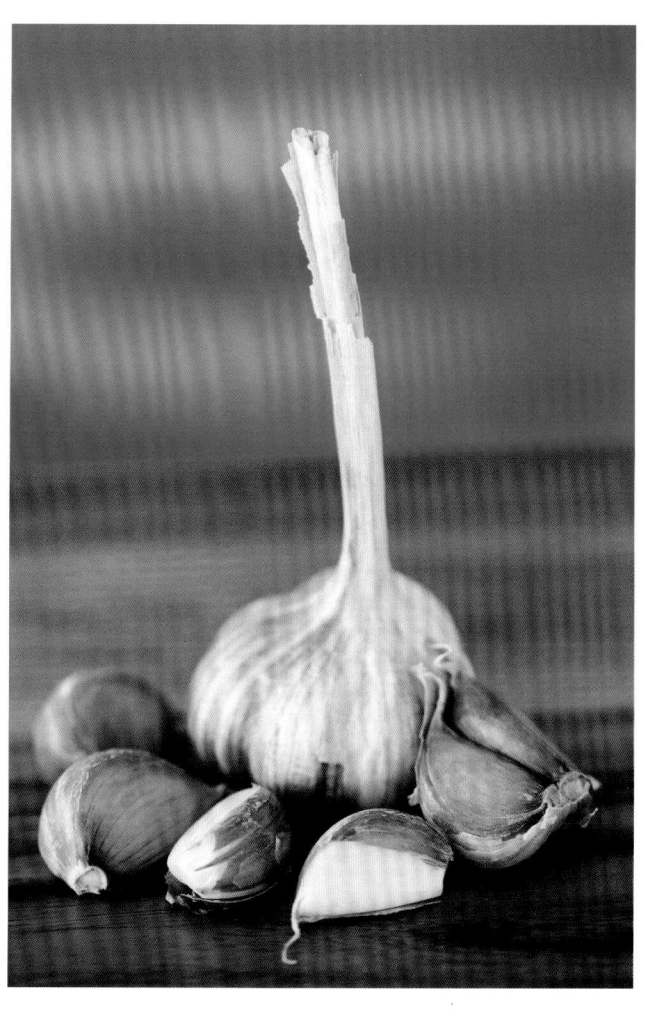

Liver

Liver is a vitamin-rich food, but also a cholesterol-rich food, that is most commonly found in the form of pâtés and sausages. Most any kind of liver provides a lot of Vitamin B6, but turkey liver provides the most, with 1.04 mg (52% RDA) in a 100gram serving, or 0.86 mg (43% RDA) in an average turkey liver. Beef liver provides 1.03 mg (51% RDA) of Vitamin B6 per 100gram serving, or 0.832 mg (42% RDA) per slice.

Fish (Tuna, Salmon, and Cod)

Fish is a heart-healthy food and a good source of protein. Yellowfin tuna provides the most Vitamin B6, with 1.04 mg (52% RDA) per 100 g serving, or 0.88 mg (44% RDA) in a 3-ounce serving. Wild caught Atlantic salmon provides 0.94 mg (47% RDA) per 100gram serving, 1.45 mg (73% RDA) in half a fillet, and 0.8 mg (40% RDA) in a 3-ounce serving. Dry cooked Pacific cod will provide 0.462 mg (23% RDA) of Vitamin B6 per 100gram serving, 0.42mg (21% RDA) in a fillet, and 0.39 mg (20% RDA) in a 3-ounce serving.

Raw Garlic

Raw garlic provides a host of health benefits, and is also a great source of Vitamin B6. Raw garlic is a great base to salad dressings, and also makes a good condiment. One hundred grams of raw garlic provides 1.235 mg (62% RDA) of Vitamin B6– that is, 1.68 (84% RDA) per cup and 0.04 mg (2% RDA) per clove or teaspoon.

Molasses and Sorghum Syrup

Molasses and sorghum syrup are high in vitamins and minerals, and make a good substitute for refined sugar and corn syrup. Molasses, also a high magnesium food, provides 0.67 mg (34% RDA) of Vitamin B6 per 100gram serving, or 2.26 mg (113% RDA) per cup, and 0.13 mg (7% RDA) per tablespoon. Sorghum syrup provides slightly less, with 0.67 mg (34% RDA) of Vitamin B6 per 100gram serving, 2.21mg (111%RDA) per cup, and 0.14 mg (7% RDA) per tablespoon.

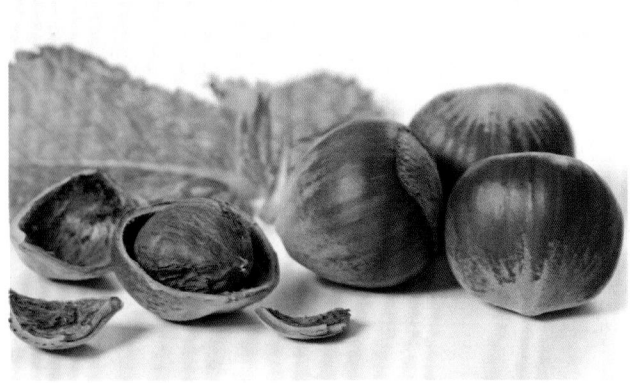

Hazelnuts or Filberts

Hazelnuts make a great snack and are also a good source of potassium and copper. Dry roasted hazelnuts provide 0.62 mg (31% RDA) of Vitamin B6 per 100gram serving, or 0.17 mg (9% RDA) per ounce.

Essential Nutrient #3: Vitamin B12

Vitamin B12 is one of the most important nutrients in the human body. It is a bright red crystalline compound that gets its color from the element cobalt, which is at its center. Vitamin B12 works with folic acid in many body processes, including synthesis of DNA, red blood cells and the insulation sheath that surrounds nerve cells and facilitates the conduction of signals to the nervous system.

Most people know of B12 as the vitamin that supports their energy levels. But there's a lot more to this vitamin than that. B12 is essential for you brain, your nervous system, your heart, your mental health and – yes – your eyesight. If you do not get enough B12, your health is going to suffer.

When it comes to sources of Vitamin B12, this vitamin is a little unusual. While most vitamins can be made from a wide variety of plants and specific animals, no plant or animal is capable of producing Vitamin B12.

The exclusive source of B12 is tiny micro-organisms such as bacteria, yeasts, molds and algae. Animals contain the microorganisms that create B12. They also eat the plants on which the B12 producing microorganisms live. In a way, B12 is similar to a probiotic. The term B12 is actually a catch-all used to describe a group of vitamins known as cobalamins.

Vitamin B12 and Vision

Scientists have only recently begun to discover the important role that Vitamin B12 plays in eye health. They have found that B12 is especially effective in helping people who suffer from age-related macular degeneration (AMD).

A 2009 study found that a mixture of Vitamin B12, B6 and folic acid reduced the risk of female study participants getting AMD by a massive 34% (72).

The randomized double-blind clinical study involved 5,442 women. All of the women already had heart disease or at least three risk factors for cardiovascular disease. Most of the women did not suffer from AMD at the beginning of the seven-year study. The researchers believed that cardiovascular disease and AMD shared common risk factors.

Another area where Vitamin B12 can assist with vision relates to optic neuropathy. The optic nerve carries vital messages to the brain. When this nerve is compromised, our vision is put in danger. Yet, one of the symptoms of Vitamin B12 deficiency is that the optic nerve becomes brittle, with a resulting decrease in central vision.

A 2012 study found that supplementation of B12, with no other changes to lifestyle or diet, put an end to the vision loss of a 68-year-old man. Not only that, but the eyesight of this man, which had been close to nonexistent, returned to a 20/20 level within a few months (73).

Think of it – *the man was on the fast track to blindness*. And there was nothing that the medical community could do to stop it. **Yet, in just a few months, supplementation with Vitamin B12 completely fixed this man's eyes!**

Another study involved three autistic children. These children were on a vegan diet, which had precipitated Vitamin B12 deficiency. As a result, they had vision problems. Yet, Vitamin B12 supplementation was able to *vastly improve the vision of all three children (74).*

Sources of Vitamin B12

The three key sources of Vitamin B12 are:

- Animal foods
- Plant foods with B12 in them (in moderation)
- Probiotics naturally present in the human gut that create B12

Animal Foods

B12 is found almost exclusively in the following animal foods:

- Liver
- Kidney

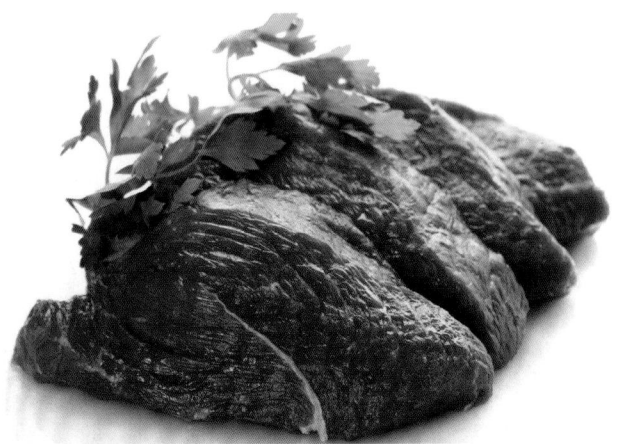

- Meat
- Fish
- Shellfish
- Meat products
- Eggs

However, the original source of Vitamin B12 in nature is bacteria. These are the only creatures who are able to manufacture this vitamin. Bivalves, such as clams, mussels and oysters, contain high levels of B12. This is because they siphon large quantities of Vitamin B12 synthesizing microorganisms.

Here are the 10 foods that are richest in Vitamin B12, based on recent research:

- Calf's liver (braised)
- Sardines
- Snapper (broiled/baked)
- Venison
- Salmon (Chinook)
- Beef tenderloin
- Lamb, roasted
- Scallops (baked/broiled)
- Shrimp (steamed/broiled)
- Halibut (baked/broiled)

Looking over this list, you'd think that we'd all be getting plenty of Vitamin B12 in our diets, right?

Wrong!

Research shows that omnivores (people who eat both animal and plant-based foods) are generally deficient in B12. A longitudinal study collected food consumption data from nine 'living food eaters' (one male, eight females) as well as vegans on two occasions, two years apart. The cross-sectional study revealed significantly lower serum Vitamin B12 concentrations in vegans compared with their omnivore counterparts.

However, the average serum B12 levels for both vegan and omnivores was way too low. A healthy serum B12 level is a minimum of 550 pmol/L. Yet, the people in the study were well below this benchmark, with the vegans having an average B12 serum reading of 193 pmol/L and the omnivores coming in at an average of 311 pmol/L.

Clearly, all of us – both vegans and omnivores – need to be taking in more Vitamin B12. People over the age of 50 are at even greater risk of deficiency. That's because our ability to absorb Vitamin B12 declines with age. Of course, so does our eyesight. The connection between the two is now clear. Getting more B12 in older age will definitely improve your eyesight.

Some of the more common symptoms of Vitamin B12 deficiency are:

- Fatigue
- Irritability
- Feeing run down
- Having no energy
- Memory loss
- Depression
- Pale skin
- Brain fog
- Burning sensations
- Muscle cramps
- Bleeding gums
- Low reflexes
- Dry eye
- Macular degeneration

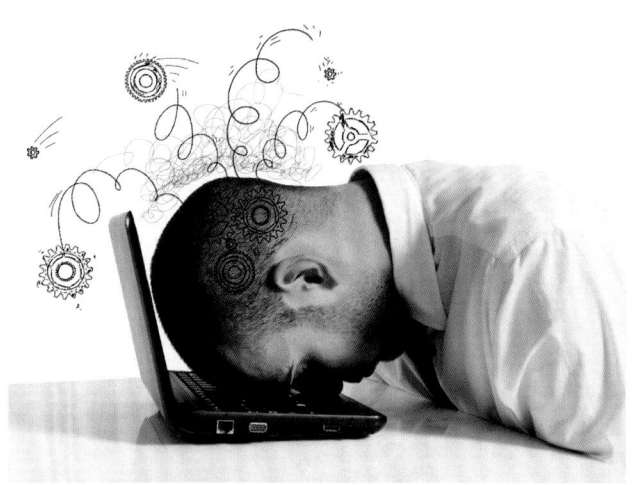

The good news is that all of those problems are completely avoidable. The recipes in our 21-day protocol will ensure that you are getting plenty of Vitamin B12 every single day.

Essential Nutrient #4: Vitamin A

Vitamin A is made up of compounds like retinol (an alcohol), and retinal (an aldehyde). Compounds of Vitamin A, like retinol and retinal, are called retinoids. Vitamin A is also made up of carotenoids, such as beta-carotene. Carotenoids are red, yellow and orange pigments that are synthesized by plants. There are hundreds of different carotenoids. However, only about 10% of these are able to form Vitamin A.

Vitamin A is a fat-soluble vitamin. That means that it is stored in your fat when you're not using it. You also need a little fat for it to work. Because your body can store Vitamin A in your liver and fatty tissue, it is possible to build up toxic amounts if you take high supplement doses.

Vitamin A is important for:

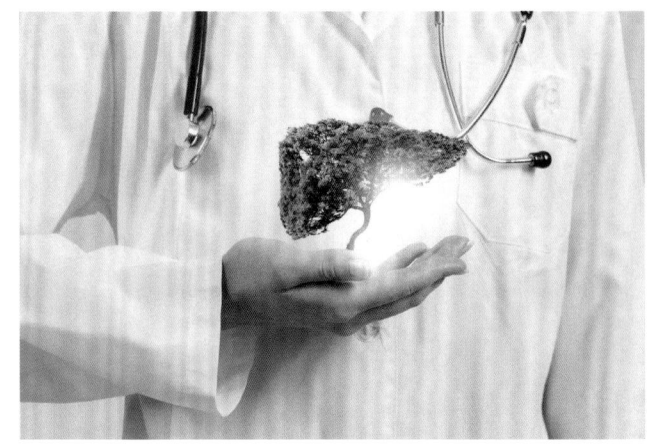

- Proper vision
- Bone growth
- Skin health
- Immune system functioning
- Growth and repair of muscle tissue
- Mucous membrane health
- Fighting and preventing infection
- Producing antibodies and white blood cells

Are You Deficient in Vitamin A?

Vitamin A deficiency among children in developing nations is the leading preventable cause of blindness. Symptoms of Vitamin A deficiency are:

- Your eyes feel uncomfortable in sunlight
- Skin becomes dry and flakey
- Acne

- Overly tingly armpits or feet
- Dry and lack-luster hair
- Peeling nails
- Weight Loss
- Diarrhea
- Insomnia
- Fatigue

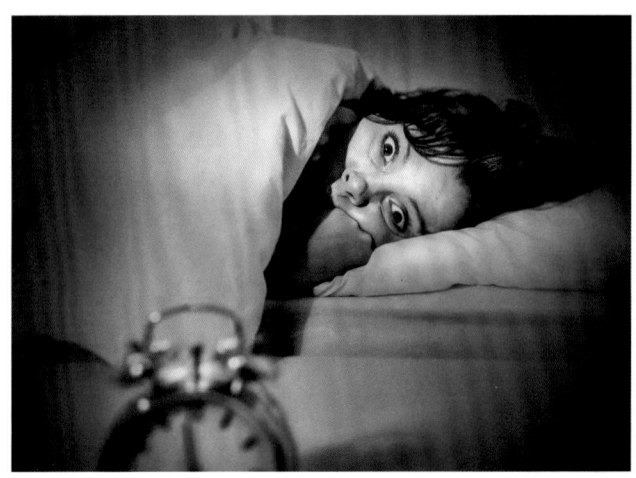

The earliest evidence of Vitamin A deficiency is night blindness. This is a condition of the eyes in which vision is normal in daylight or other strong light but is abnormally weak or completely lost at night or in dim light. It also leads to dry eye, which is characterized by abnormal dryness in the conjunctiva and cornea. This results in inflammation and ridge formation.

Vitamin A and Vision

Retinol breaks down into retinyl ester. These are then broken apart to form 11-Cis-Retinol. In turn, this is oxidized to form 11-Cis-Retinal. 11-Cisr-Retinal then moves into the rod cells, and then forms and bonds to a protein called Opsin. This creates a visual pigment called Rhodopsin.

Rhodopsin is essential in night vision. That is because it has the ability to detect very small amounts of light. The Rhodopsin is catalyzed into All-Trans-Retinol and released as a signal to the optic nerve. This signal is then conveyed to the brain, where it is comprehended as vision. Consuming Vitamin A puts more Rhodopsin in the vision cycle. The result is improved night vision.

Vitamin A and Light

Whenever you expose your eyes to light, you use up Vitamin A. So, whenever you are outside in the sunlight, your body is processing Vitamin A. It's the same thing when you're staring at a computer screen or reading a book or watching the TV screen. If you do these things a lot, you may have a Vitamin A deficiency.

A sure sign of deficiency is that you take a long time to adjust from outside light to inside light. Night blindness, finding it extremely difficult to drive at night, burning and pain in the eyes and having to wear dark glasses during the day are all signs of acute Vitamin A deficiency.

Vitamin A and Mucus

Mucus membranes line your body cavities, including the nose, throat, lungs, middle ear, urinary tract and gall bladder. Mucus membranes constantly secrete a fluid that prevents bacteria from attacking these areas of your body. When you don't have enough Vitamin A in your body, the fluid dries up, providing an opening for mucus to attack your body.

Vitamin A and Infection

Vitamin A plays an important role in the immune system. As such, it is an effective infection fighter. The skin and cells that line the digestive tract, urinary tract and airways protect the body as the first line of defense against infections. The retinol and metabolic substances in Vitamin A are essential to

the development of white blood cells, which play a major role in preventing infection.

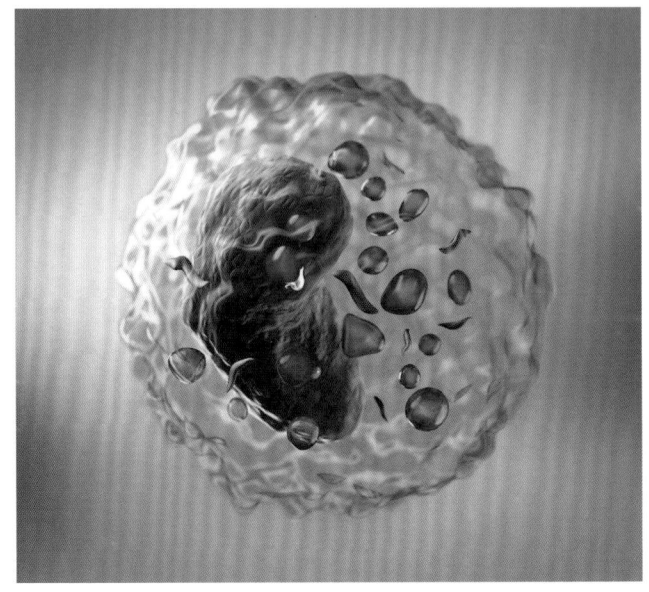

The major regulatory cells in the immune system, T-Lymphocytes, are also created by the Vitamin A compounds retinoids and carotenoids.

If you are lacking in Vitamin A, you will be at risk of infection in your:

- Respiratory system
- Kidneys
- Eyes
- Middle ear
- Sinuses
- Intestines
- Reproductive organs

Best Sources of Vitamin A

Animal food sources are good places to get your Vitamin A. Foods like cold-water fish (such as salmon), liver, and egg yolks are great sources of Vitamin A.

Your body has the ability to convert beta-carotene into Vitamin A. Your best sources of beta-carotene are plants, green leafy vegetables and any vegetable with a yellow or orange pigment.

The best sources of beta-carotene are:

- Carrots
- Squash
- Cantaloupes

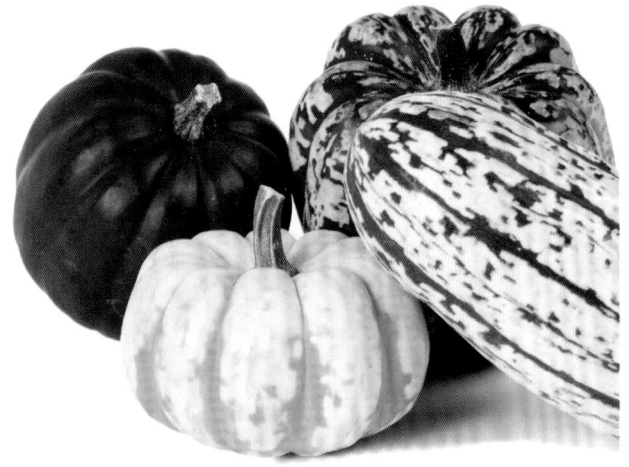

How Much?

The amount of Vitamin A that you need depends on your lifestyle. If you spend a lot of time in front of a computer screen or out in direct sunlight, you will need more of it than someone who spends a lot of time in darkness. That being said, the average dose is 50,000 units per day.

People with gastrointestinal conditions may not be able to properly absorb Vitamin A.

In contrast to preformed Vitamin A, the carotenoids in Vitamin A are not toxic. The body can form Vitamin A from carotenoids in the body like beta-carotene. This natural Vitamin A is extremely unlikely to damage your body. However, the preformed Vitamin A found in supplements can have negative effects when taken in large doses. Many supplements include three times the recommended daily allowance of Vitamin A.

It is better to get Vitamin A through natural foods than in supplemental form.

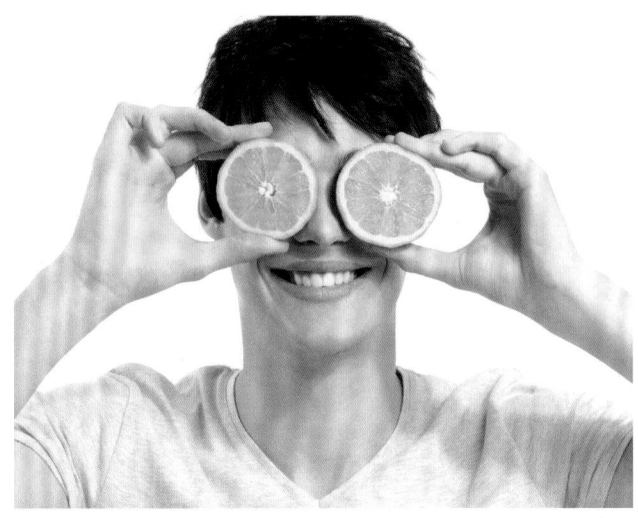

Essential Nutrient #5: Vitamin C

Widely known as an effective treatment for common colds and flu, Vitamin C is actually one of the most important nutrients needed by the body. As a health-promoting and cancer-fighting antioxidant, it plays the role of protector by preventing cell damage caused by free radicals, protecting your eyes from the effects of macular degeneration.

Vitamin C and the Eyes

Vitamin C is a water-soluble antioxidant. As such, it protects your body fluids, including saliva, blood, intercellular fluids, lymph **fluids and the fluids that surround your eyes**.

The watery fluid in your eyes between the cornea and the iris is called the aqueous humor. This vital liquid gives shape to the eye. It also protects and nourishes the eye. It just so happens that aqueous humor contains very high levels of Vitamin C. The levels are even higher than that in the blood. In order to keep the eye well-nourished to protect it from the effects of free radicals, it is essential that we keep those Vitamin C levels in the aqueous humor high.

Specifically, taking in plenty of Vitamin C will help to protect your eyes from…

- Cataracts
- Glaucoma
- Macular Degeneration

A study out of Tufts University showed that women who took 362 mg or more of Vitamin C had a 57% lower risk of developing cataracts by the age of 60 when compared to women who had a daily intake of less than 140 mg of Vitamin C (75).

Another study, this time out of researchers from King's College London, analyzed data from 1,000 pairs of female twins in order to identify what factors are the most important in warding off cataracts. They were especially interested in the role that Vitamin C plays. They also analyzed the opaqueness of the women's lenses at the age of 60, and then 10 years later.

The women who took in more Vitamin C-rich foods saw a reduction of cataract progression by 33%. Study author Christopher Hammond, M.D., FRCOphth, professor of ophthalmology, commented…

While we cannot totally avoid developing cataracts, we may be able to delay their onset and keep them from worsening significantly by eating a diet rich in vitamin C (76).

A 2003 study out of Duke University in Durham, North Carolina, compared the effects of Vitamin C supplementation on the development of diabetic retinopathy (the most common diabetic eye disease). The researchers saw significant improvement in the key markers of eye health. The lead author of the study wrote…

Vitamin supplementation suppressed leukocyte adhesion and thus endothelial dysfunction, associated with increase in iris blood flow perfusion in diabetes. The antioxidant Vitamin C may be a therapeutic agent for preventing diabetic retinopathy (77).

A study by scientists at the Oregon Health and Science University, published in the *Journal of Neuroscience*, discovered that previously unknown cells in the eyes need Vitamin C in order to work properly. Study co-author Henrique von Gersdorff, PhD, commented…

We found that cells in the retina need to be 'bathed' in relatively high doses of vitamin C, inside and out, to function properly. Because the retina is part of the central nervous system, this suggests there's likely an important role for vitamin C throughout our brains, to a degree we had not realized before (78).

Our brains contain special receptors, known as GABA-type receptors. Their job is to help modulate speedy communication between the cells in the brain. GABA receptors act like an inhibitory brake on exhibitory neurons in the brain. The Oregon study found that when Vitamin C was removed, the GABA-type retinal cells stopped functioning properly.

Researchers don't fully understand the role of Vitamin C in the brain. They do know that when we deprive ourselves of Vitamin C, it stays in the brain longer than anywhere else. This could have relevance to another eye disease – glaucoma. This condition is caused by the malfunctioning of nerve cells on the retina. These cells become over excited due to this malfunctioning.

'For example, maybe a vitamin C-rich diet could be neuroprotective for the retina – for people who are especially prone to glaucoma,' Dr. von Gersdorff said. *'This is speculative and there is much to learn. But this research provides some important insights and will lead to the generation of new hypotheses and potential treatment strategies.'*

Best Sources of Vitamin C

While supplementing with Vitamin C capsules has become very popular, it is always best to get your Vitamin C from natural, whole food sources.

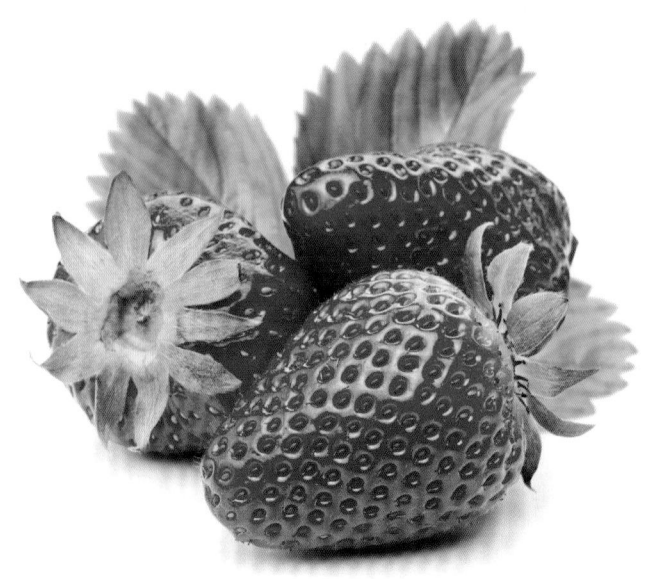

Some great sources of Vitamin C are:

- Citrus Fruits
- Tomatoes
- Green Leafy Vegetables
- Broccoli
- Blackcurrants
- Strawberries
- Blueberries
- Raw Cabbage

Essential Nutrient #6: Zinc

Zinc is a mineral that benefits you across the board. Whether you are interested in improving your vision, losing weight, fortifying your immune system or even building muscle, zinc needs to form a key part of your nutritional arsenal.

Zinc is actually a cofactor for more than 500 biochemical reactions in the body. The majority of this activity takes place in the brain; that is why zinc is recognized as an important nootropic. All aspects of your mental health, including memory, mood, focus and the senses, are reliant on zinc. Even our taste buds are zinc dependent, with loss of taste being a major sign of zinc deficiency.

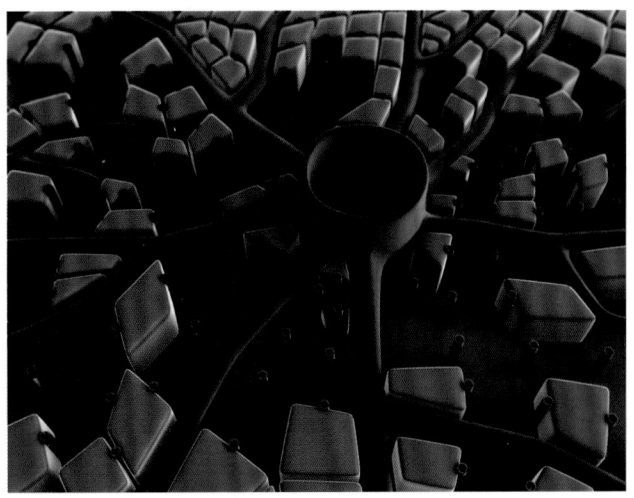

Zinc and Vision

The majority of people with vision problems end up being zinc deficient. Zinc plays the vital role of bringing Vitamin A from the liver to the retina, where it produces melanin – the protective pigment in the eye. As a result, zinc concentrations in the eye are very high, especially in the retina and the choroid, which is the tissue layer that lies beneath the retina.

Taking in more zinc will help people who are at risk of age-related macular degeneration (AMD). The Age-Related Eye Disease Study (AREDS), which was sponsored by the National Eye Institute, showed definitively that AMD is related to nutrition. The study revealed that people who are at high risk of AMD can slow the progression of the disease by 25% by taking 40-80 mg of zinc daily. Visual acuity loss can be reduced by 19% by taking in the same amount.

A study that was published in the *African Journal of Food, Agricultural, Nutrition and Development* revealed that zinc deficiency was implicated in the high incidence of cataract formation. Cataract formation is more common in countries where there is prolonged exposure to sunlight, leading to a greater level of ultraviolet light penetration. Zinc is able to protect the lens of the eye from oxidative damage (79) (80).

Our bodies do not produce the zinc that we require, which means that we must take it in through our diet.

Zinc Deficiency

Zinc is one of the most essential nutrients that supports the immune system. Yet, the experts tell us that as many as two billion people around the world are zinc deficient. And, don't think that zinc deficiency is just a problem in developing countries. In fact, about 12% of Americans do not consume enough zinc. They fail to reach the minimum RDA for zinc and could be at risk of a zinc deficiency.

So, how do you find out if your zinc intake is too low? The common symptoms of zinc deficiency are:

- Lack of appetite
- Moodiness
- A less keen sense of taste or smell

Zinc deficiency is especially common among vegans and vegetarians. Many vegetarians consume grains, which contain high levels of phytic acid. Phytic acid greatly reduces the bioavailability of zinc. Zinc from plant sources is not as well absorbed because animal foods do not contain phytic acid.

As with all minerals, the ideal way to get more zinc is by eating healthy foods rather than taking a supplement. The following foods are high in zinc:

- Green peas (in moderation)
- Beans (in moderation)
- Mushrooms
- Spinach
- Sea vegetables
- Pumpkin seeds
- Oysters
- Organic, grass fed beef
- Organic liver

You will notice that most of these zinc sources come from plants. However, there are things that you can do to increase the body's absorption of zinc, despite the fact that the plants contain phytic acid. You can soak beans and

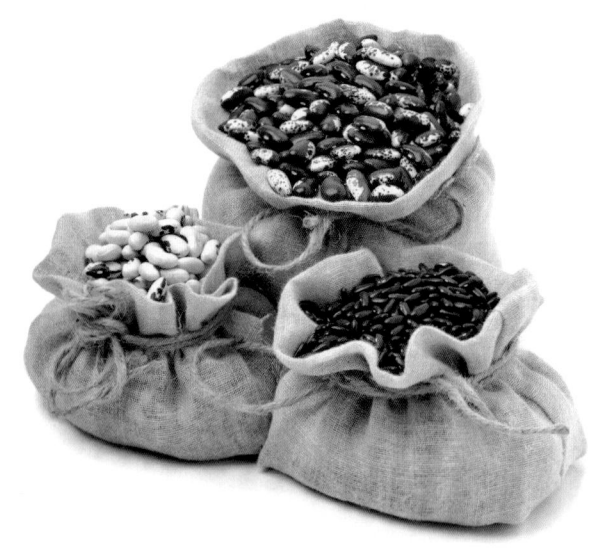

seeds in water for several hours before cooking them. This helps to remove the phytic acid that binds to the zinc and other vital minerals. The best temperature to soak these foods in is about 140 degrees, and they should be soaked for about three hours. Doing this can actually remove about half of the phytic acid.

Eating leavened as opposed to unleavened grains (in moderation) will also reduce your phytic acid intake.

A major cause of zinc deficiency is stress. Ironically, people who regularly exercise are also prone to zinc deficiency because you lose zinc when you sweat. But that's no reason to stop exercising – just be sure to get plenty of zinc-rich foods in your diet.

Being exposed to environmental toxins, such as bisphenol A (BPA) plastics will prevent you from absorbing zinc.

Perhaps the greatest contributor to zinc deficiency, however, has to do with the inferior quality of the soil we grow our food in. You may have never given much thought to it, but the soil that we take for granted is actually a living ecosystem. In it, dead organic matter forms the basis of an intricate food web. One key nutrient that we get from soil is zinc – or we used to, anyway.

The problem is that mineral fertilizers, along with such farming practices as mechanical digging, play havoc with the fungi in soil. These fungi are critical in helping plants absorb such minerals from the soil as zinc.

The result of all of this is that even when we eat traditionally zinc-rich plant foods, such as cereal grains, we are not getting the amount of zinc that our ancestors got – because our soil is zinc depleted.

That is why plants that are produced under organic farming conditions contain more vitamins and minerals and are the smarter choice – especially when you are trying to improve your eyesight.

CHAPTER ELEVEN

THE 10 BERRIES THAT CAN HELP SAVE YOUR VISION

Our analysis of the list of vision superfoods that Bunji handed me years go showed that the Aboriginals of Australia had a diet rich in a variety of berries. These proved fantastic for their eyesight. The main reason was that they were very high in antioxidants.

Scientists have recently discovered that berries are among the most powerful disease fighting foods on the planet. That's because they are packed with antioxidants, which give them their vibrant colors. The antioxidants in berries have been shown to lower the risks of a number of cancers, in addition to helping with poor memory and countering the effects of old age (81).

Berries are also a great source of dietary fiber.

Although berries are seasonal, frozen berries contain all of the health-giving benefits of fresh, and are available all

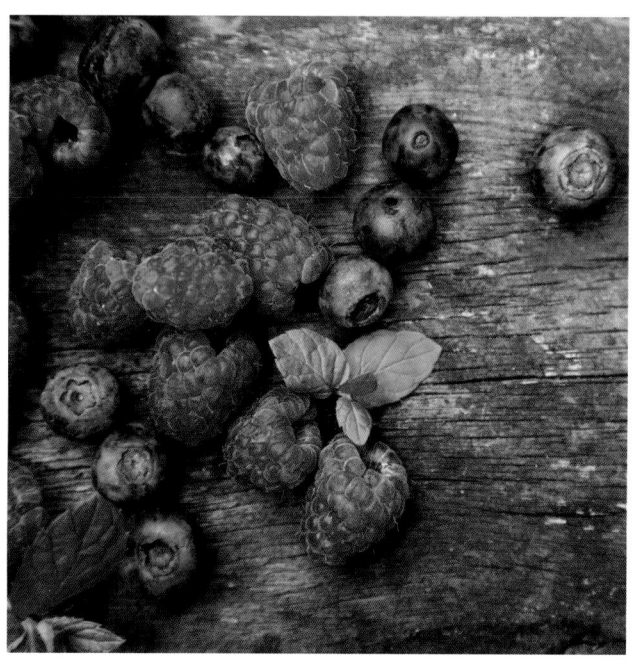

year round.

As we discovered in Chapter Two, free radical damage is the main culprit in deteriorating eyesight. The antioxidants that are packed inside of berries are a key line of defense against this free radical damage. In this chapter, we zoom in on 10 berries that you can pick up at your local supermarket in order to help preserve your vision.

Blueberries

According to the USDA Human Nutritional Center, blueberries rank number one in antioxidant benefits compared to 40 other fruits and vegetables. These antioxidants are your first line of defense against the ravaging effects of free radicals on your eyesight.

The total antioxidant capacity of blueberries is twice as much as spinach and three times as much as oranges. This extraordinary fruit is also rich in pectin, a soluble fiber that has been shown to be effective in lowering cholesterol.

Berries also have a high flavonoid count. Flavonoids are believed to have a beneficial effect on the cardiovascular system. Blueberries, in particular, have a high flavonoid count (82).

Blueberries have also been shown to improve vascular circulation in the tiny blood vessels in your eyes. As a result, your eyes are better able to adjust to the light, making this berry especially beneficial for improving night vision.

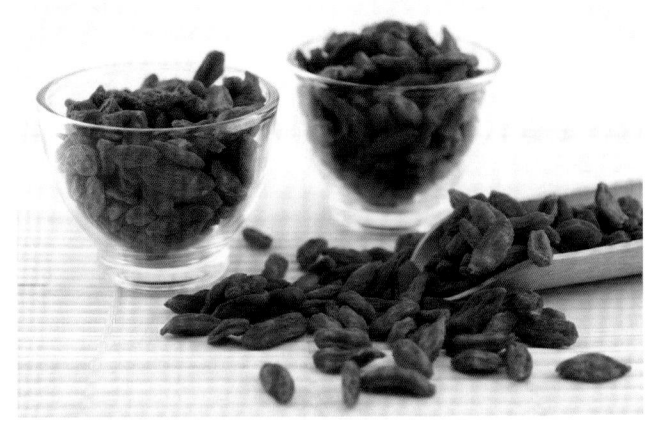

Goji Berry

Recently, a super berry has been revealed to the Western world; it provides the antioxidant effects of other berries **multiplied by a factor of 5**. This incredible food has the most antioxidants of any food yet discovered. It's grown at one of the highest altitudes on earth; the distant mountains of Tibet.

It is the **GOJI BERRY**.

Goji berries are causing a sensation in the nutritional world, with researchers calling them the Rolls Royce of berries.

The Goji berry is especially rich in zeaxanthin and beta carotene, two of the most important antioxidants for eye health. That makes them an essential weapon in fighting against the devastating effects that free radicals have on the macula (83).

Grapes

Grapes are very rich in antioxidants. They contain high levels of flavonoids, phenolic acid and resveratrol, all of which are invaluable phytonutrients known as 'polyphenols.' They are also rich in vitamins A, B1, B2, B6 and C. This combination of compounds provides a powerful defense against the oxidative stress that is so detrimental to the eyes (84).

A recent study out of the University of Miami found that grapes were an exceptionally effective counter to the damaging effects of free radicals on photoreceptors in the retina. The study involved feeding either freeze-dried whole grape powder or a standard research control diet to mice. Both

retinal structure and function were preserved in the grape eating group. Retinal thickness was maintained, and the quantity and amount of photoreceptor activity was maintained despite intense levels of oxidative stress. In the standard diet group, the retinas were extensively damaged as a result of oxidative stress.

Lead researcher professor Abigail Hackman said:

Adding grapes to the diet actually preserved retinal health in the presence of oxidative stress in this study. These results are very exciting and build on the growing evidence that suggests a very real benefit for grape consumption (85).

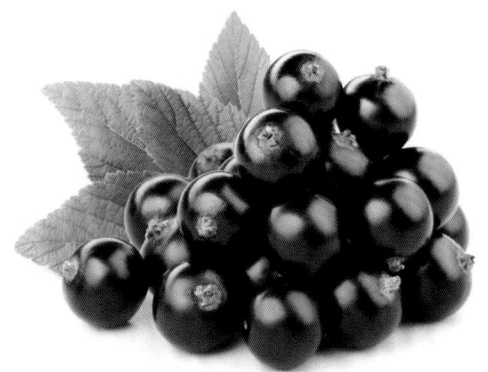

Blackcurrant

Blackcurrants are a very rich source of anthocyanins, the compounds that give

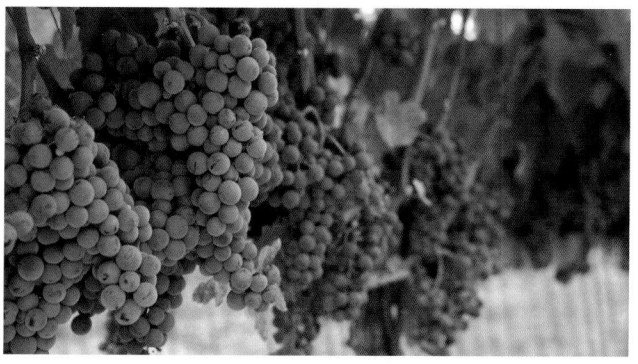

them their dark color. Anthocyanins are able to fight against the free radical damage that affects our eyes.

One study revealed that blackcurrants can also have a profound effect on the ability of the eye to adjust to changes in light. In the study, participants were given the equivalent of one tablespoon of blackcurrant juice daily. Results saw that dark adaptation was increased by 50%, while visual fatigue was decreased by up to 200% (86).

Studies have also shown that blackcurrants are a powerful defense against glaucoma. In one study,

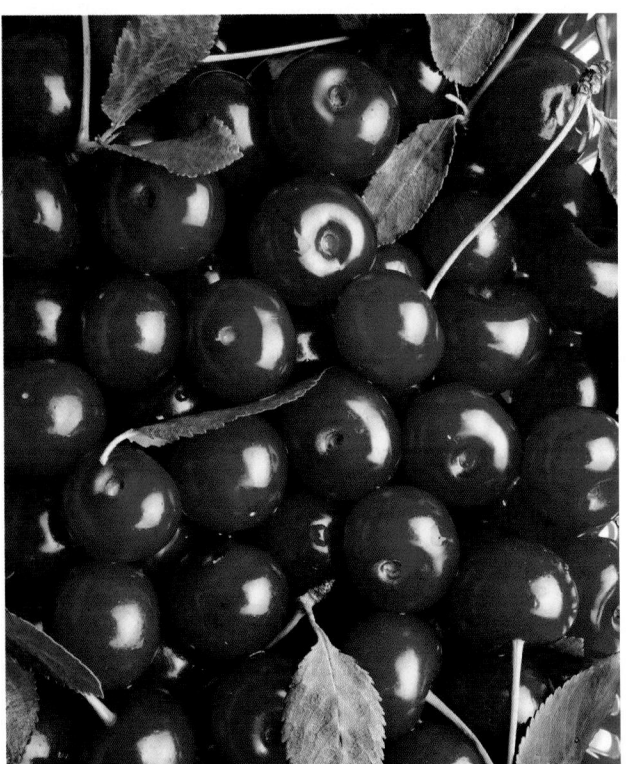

participants were given 50 mg of blackcurrant juice per day for six months. All subjects had a marked improvement in blood flow through the veins in the eyes. This significantly improved their eyesight (87).

In another study, the effects of blackcurrant on intraocular pressure was examined. Daily consumption of 50 mg of blackcurrant anthocyanins significantly decreased intraocular pressure and significantly decreased visual field deterioration (88).

Blackberry

Blackberries are rich in antioxidant Vitamins A and C, both of which are vital to eye health. They are also rich in lutein, which forms a protective pigment behind the retina. In addition, blackberries are packed with phenolic acids, which are powerful antioxidant compounds.

Cherries

Cherries are a fantastic natural defense against the damaging effects of ultraviolet radiation on the eyes. This is thanks to the natural chemical that gives them their color – anthocyanins.

Anthocyanins are used by the body to produce essential amino acids. As antioxidants, anthocyanins protect the cells of the eyes from the damaging effects of ultraviolet radiation.

Cherries also contain a lot of beta-carotene, the precursor to Vitamin A. In fact, there is 19 times more beta-carotene in cherries than in blueberries!

Cranberry

Cranberries are extremely high in all of the key vitamins we have identified for improved eye health, including:

- Vitamin A
- Vitamin C
- Vitamin B6
- Vitamin B12

They are also packed with manganese, which is a potent fighter against free radicals. Cranberries have very high levels of flavonoids and antioxidants, making them a powerful defense against the oxidative stress that leads to vision loss.

Bilberry

Bilberries are full of anthocyanosides, which are compounds with strong antioxidative properties. Bilberries look much like blueberries, but have a much darker skin. That is due to the anthocyanosides. Because of their antioxidative properties, bilberries have a powerful effect on the tiny blood vessels in the eyes.

It is reputed that, during the Battle of Britain, British Royal Air Force pilots ate bilberry jam before a flight to enhance their night vision.

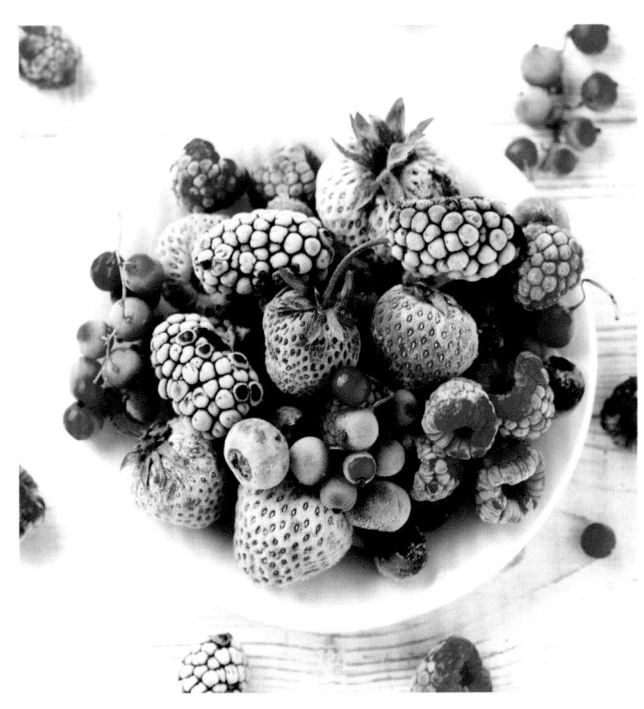

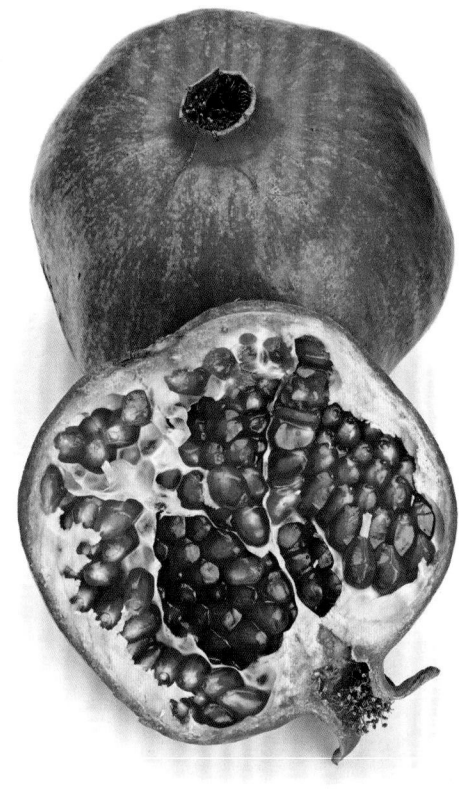

Pomegranate

Pomegranates are rich in punicalagins, which are powerful antioxidants. In fact, the antioxidant level is even higher than in blueberries, cranberries or oranges. This is largely due to the high levels of polyphenols, which will directly combat free radical damage to the eyes.

Pomegranates are also a great source of the B vitamins and Vitamin C, which are vital for eye health. They also contain a lot of beta-carotene, the precursor to Vitamin A.

Pomegranates also have the ability to help the body produce a compound called Rhodopsin, the eye pigmentation that helps you to adjust from light to dark conditions, as well as improve night vision.

Strawberry

As well as being one of the most delicious berries out there, strawberries are an excellent source of Vitamins C, B6 and B12, as well as flavonoids. They also contain high levels of manganese and folate. The compounds in strawberries help relieve ocular pressure, which promotes proper eyesight and relieves eye strain.

Strawberries are also rich in potassium, which improves the circulation to the small blood vessels in the eyes. This also helps relieve eye pressure (and the resulting pain).

CHAPTER **TWELVE**

THE TOXIC FOODS THAT YOU NEED TO AVOID FOR YOUR EYE'S SAKE

So far, we've discovered that there are certain foods that will go directly to your eyes to fight the damaging effects of free radicals. However, there are also foods that you absolutely need to stay away from in order to protect your vision. These very common household foods are more than likely lurking around in your pantry or fridge. Until you get rid of them, you will be minimizing the effects of all of the good things that you are putting into your body.

Here are the top five foods that you need to nix in order to protect your eyesight.

(1) Margarine

It probably comes as no surprise that margarine is bad for you. But did you know that it can negatively impact on your vision?

Two major US studies revealed that a higher risk of macular degeneration occurred in people who ate larger quantities of vegetable fat, with margarine being a main contributor. The researchers put this down to the high amounts of trans fatty acids contained in the margarine. Trans fats lead to oxidative damage, with the result that there is an increased amount of free radical damage in the retina (89) (90).

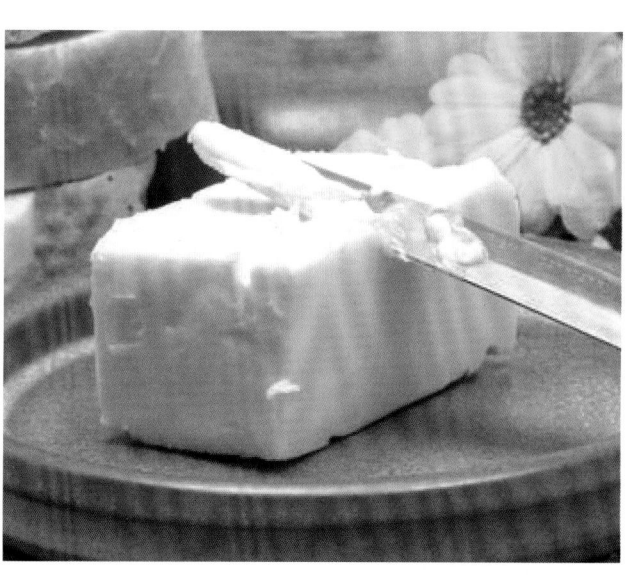

An Australian study showed that a diet that was high in processed fats like margarine brought a fourfold risk of blindness. The lead researcher of the study, Professor Paul Beaumont, commented...

The oils that you eat become part of your eye, but normally they're used and flushed out. Researchers believe the eye finds it particularly difficult to biodegrade vegetable oils. They end up blocking the eye's cells and causing macular degeneration (91).

Margarine is especially high in trans fats. These are manmade fats that cannot be absorbed by the human body. Their only purpose is to keep products on the shelf longer.

Margarine was originally manufactured to fatten turkeys. But the plan backfired – all the turkeys died! What could they do with this product that they'd poured all of their money into?

The product was originally white and had no food appeal. So, they decided to add yellow coloring to it and market it as an alternative to butter.

Butter and margarine both have the same number of calories. Butter has slightly more saturated fat at seven grams, compared to five grams from margarine. But that hardly tells the story.

Eating margarine can increase the risk of heart disease by 53 percent in women compared to butter, according to a recent Harvard medical study. It also increases the risk of cancer up to five times.

When you eat butter, it increases the absorption of many other nutrients in your food. And then you have the alternative to butter – **margarine is but one molecule away from being plastic.**

Margarine also shares 27 ingredients with paint.

If you want to find out how bad margarine really is, simply place an open container of the stuff in a dark corner of your basement and leave it for a couple of days. You will find that no bugs will dare go near it. Nor will the margarine rot or grow tiny micro-organisms. Why?

Because it has absolutely no nutritional value.

Bottom line: stay away from margarine.

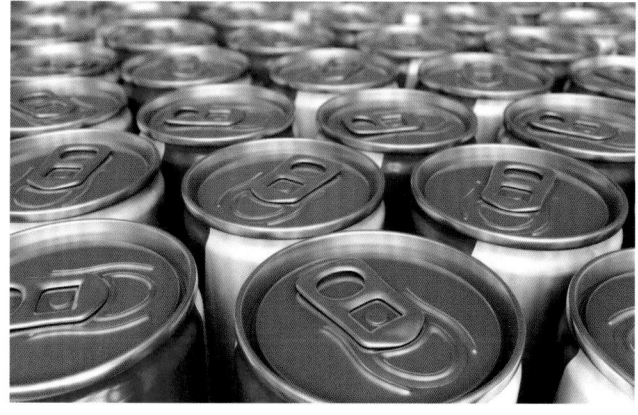

(2)   Sugary Drinks

Sugary drinks have a lot to answer for. As well as making us fat, slow and lethargic, they are also causing us to lose our eyesight. The main reason, of course, is the massive amount of sugar they contain. The sugars that are added to soft drinks have absolutely no nutritional value.

Recent research has shown a clear link between the consumption of sugary soft drinks and serious eye conditions. The AREDS study results revealed that people who were at risk of developing age-related macular degeneration (AMD) would benefit by drastically reducing their consumption of sugary drinks.

High concentrations of sugar in the lens of the eye leads to damage in the proteins of the retina and causes the clumping that results in the formation of cataracts. Consumption of high-sugar drinks has also been shown to aggravate the symptoms of dry eye.

When we drink high-sugar soft drinks, we get a sugar spike in the blood. This brings far too much glucose to the eye, which hampers its ability to properly make use of that energy. The excess causes swelling and cataract formation (92).

(3)   High Fat Cuts of Meat

You need to consume a certain amount of red meat for your eye health. Red meat is high in zinc, which, as we've already discovered, is a key nutrient for optimal vision. However, when you eat too much red meat that is high in fat, you will actually be causing damage to your eyes.

A study out of the Centre for Eye Research in Melbourne, Australia, found that people who ate red meat

10 times or more per week had a 50% higher risk of developing macular degeneration when compared to people who ate lean cuts of red meat a maximum of four times per week. It was also shown that people who ate a lot of sausage and salami had a much higher risk of macular degeneration. In comparison, those who ate chicken did not have an increased risk of macular degeneration (93).

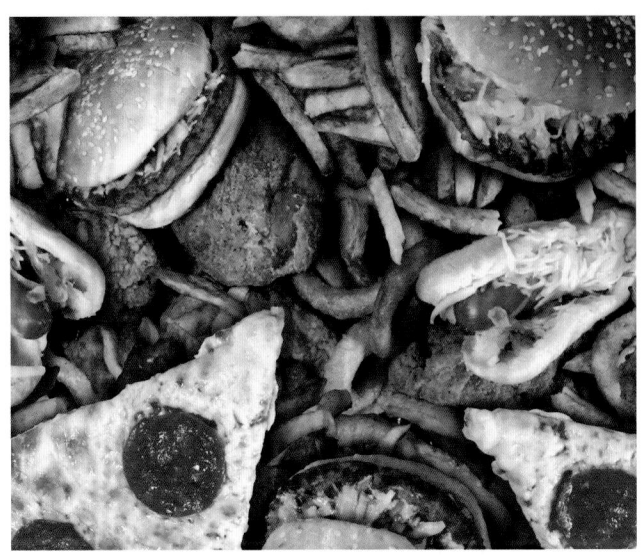

High-fat cuts of red meat result in increased fatty acids being transported to the tiny blood vessels in the eyes, clogging them up and reducing vision.

In order to ensure that your love of red meat doesn't impact your vision, limit yourself to four red meat based main meals per week. Choose lean cuts and keep your portions to the size of your closed fist.

(4)   Junk Food

Junk food isn't only making you fat – it's also causing you to go blind! According to a study conducted by researchers at the Massachusetts Eye and Ear Infirmary, fat-filled junk foods significantly increase the risk of developing age-related macular degeneration. The study involved 349 subjects between the ages of 55 and 80. They all had advanced stages of age-related macular degeneration. Their diets were rich in French fries, pies, cakes, burgers and cookies (94).

The high levels of fat that you consume when you eat a high junk food diet will damage the blood vessels and capillaries that transport nutrients and oxygen to the retina of your eyes. When you can't get these vital nutrients, your eyes are literally being starved of what they need to function properly.

(5)   Breakfast Cereals

Breakfast cereals are packed with massive amounts of sugar. They are also loaded with GMOs that are toxic to the body. Just as when you drink a lot of sugary soft drinks, all of that sugar overpowers your eyes, leading to dry eye, swelling and cataracts.

Removing breakfast cereals from your diet is a necessary step on your way to optimum eye health.

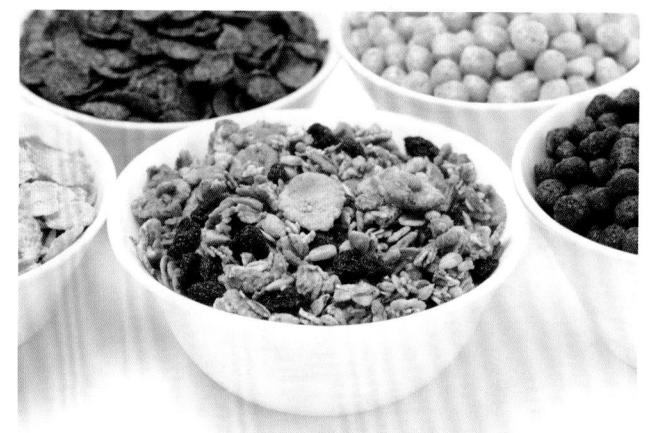

CHAPTER **THIRTEEN**

YOUR 21 DAY SMOOTHIE PROTOCOL

OK – so, the Aboriginal people of Australia didn't actually drink smoothies!

But that doesn't mean that you shouldn't. By adding the special ingredients that we've already uncovered from our examination of the Aboriginal diet, you'll be able to create delicious smoothies that will provide your body with a power-packed energy boost. Better still, each mouthful will be helping you to a diabetes-free future.

By combining these ingredients to defeat free radicals and reclaim your eyesight in the form of a smoothie, you'll be able to get all of the nutrients you need in one, easy to consume meal.

The greatest source of lutein and zeaxanthin is green leafy vegetables, which is why they form the foundation of our smoothie protocol.

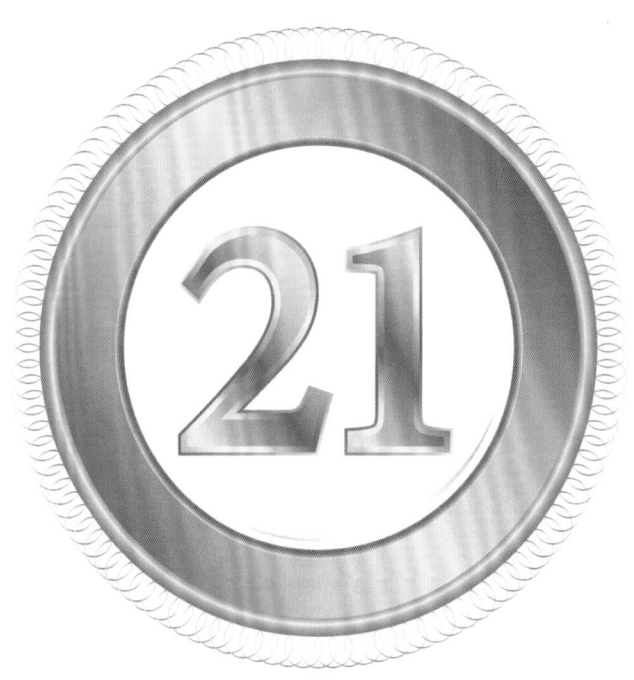

The Western world has seen a decline in vegetable consumption over the last 20 years. The preference for fast foods, lack of time and general life pressures have seen the humble lettuce, broccoli, cucumber and parsnip relegated to the vegetable bin while people pig out on pizza and French fries.

The smoothie has the power to bring back vegetables, along with juices in a super convenient, delicious way. In this guide, you will discover 21 smoothie recipes that will greatly boost your vision, while also giving your body the vitamins it needs to operate optimally.

How to Implement the Protocol

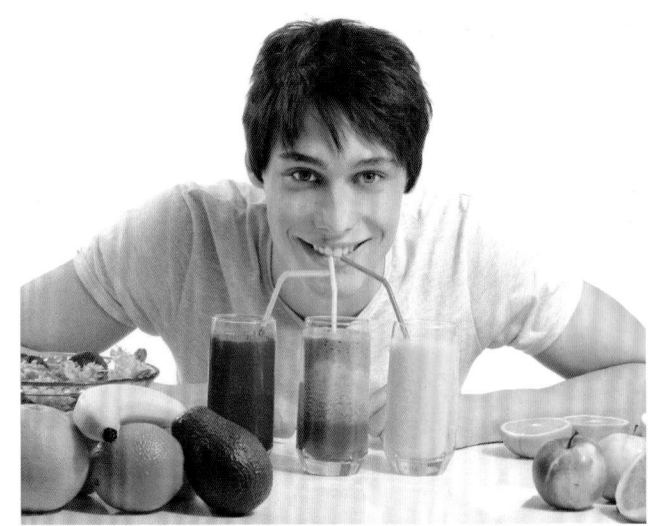

1) Have a smoothie three times per day following the Seven-Day Guidelines provided in the following pages. Enjoy your three daily smoothies as snacks between meals – you can also use one of your daily smoothies as a meal replacement if you are trying to lose weight. After completing the seven days, repeat the protocol until you get the results you desire. Continue the protocol for a full 21 days to achieve the best results.

2) Do not change your normal meal patterns, apart from implementing the guidelines in Chapter Eleven about cutting out toxic foods.

3) If you are trying to lose weight in addition to improving your eye health, you may opt to have your shake as a meal replacement for one meal each day.

June 18 →1

THE SMOOTHIES

DAY 1 SMOOTHIE # 1
LIFTED BLACKBERRY SMOOTHIE

Key Vision Nutrients (per serving):

Lutein
Zeaxanthin
Omega-3

Prep Time: 30 seconds

Serves: 2

Ingredients:

- 1 cup frozen blackberries
- 2 small bananas - peeled
- 2 tablespoons coconut cream
- 2 tablespoons maca powder
- 3 ice cubes

Steps:

1. Place all ingredients in blender and blend on high until smooth.

Nutrition Data: 175 calories, 4.3g fat, 33.8g carbs, 3.4g protein, 7.8g fiber, 17.4g sugar, 4mg sodium

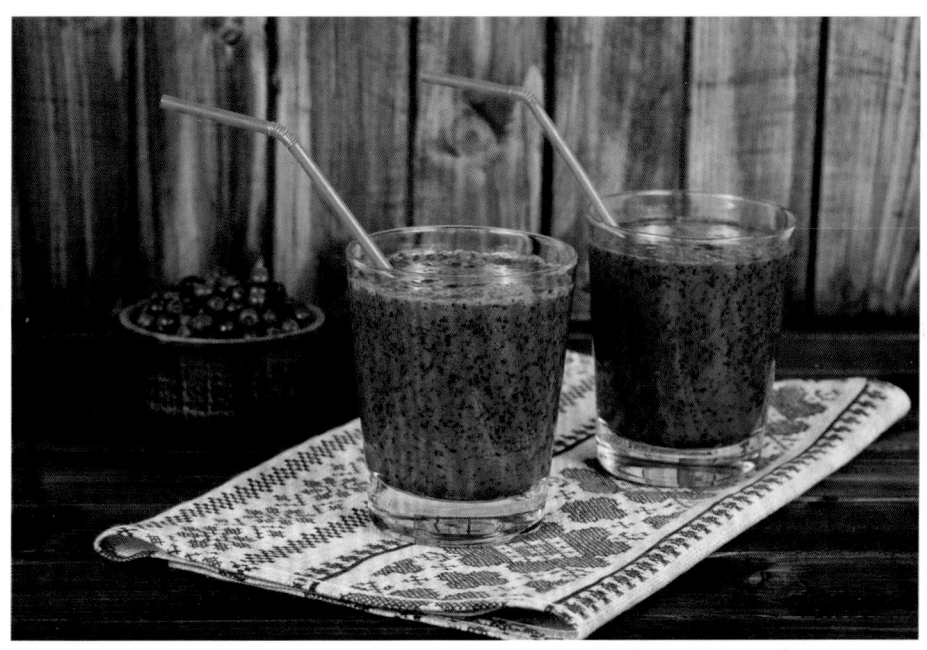

June 19 - 2

DAY 1 SMOOTHIE # 2
VEGGIE MIX

Key Vision Nutrients (per serving):

Lutein

Zeaxanthin

Vitamin B6

Vitamin B12

Prep Time: 30 seconds

Serves: 1

Ingredients:

- 1 small red beet, chopped
- 1 small carrot, chopped
- 1 small green apple (cored and chopped)
- 1 small pear (chopped)
- 1 cup chopped kale
- 2 cups water
- 2 tablespoons lemon juice (fresh)
- 2 tablespoons ginger (grated)

Steps:

1. Blend all the ingredients together.

Nutrition Data: 330 calories, 1.6g fat, 79.9g carbs, 6g protein, 14.9g fiber, 46.2g sugar, 134mg sodium

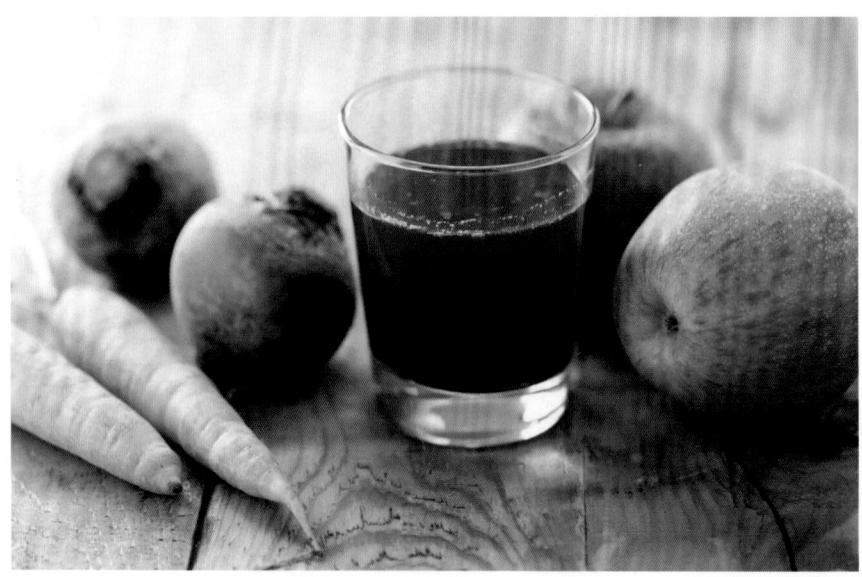

DAY 1 SMOOTHIE # 3
LEAN GREEN MACHINE

Key Vision Nutrients (per serving):

Lutein
Zeaxanthin
Vitamin B12
Zinc

Prep Time: 30 seconds

Serves: 1

Ingredients:

- 2 cups chopped spinach
- ½ cup chopped broccoli
- 1 cup chopped kale
- 1 cup chopped cucumber
- 1 tablespoon chia seeds
- ¼ cup chopped pineapple
- ¼ cup chopped mango
- 1 small carrot, chopped
- Ginger (as much as you can handle)
- 1-2 cups water

Steps:

1. Blend the spinach and water together first.
2. Once the mixture is creamy, add the remaining ingredients and blend for 45 seconds.

Nutrition Data: 208 calories, 5.8g fat, 39.8g carbs, 9.8g protein, 11.7g fiber, 15g sugar, 129mg sodium

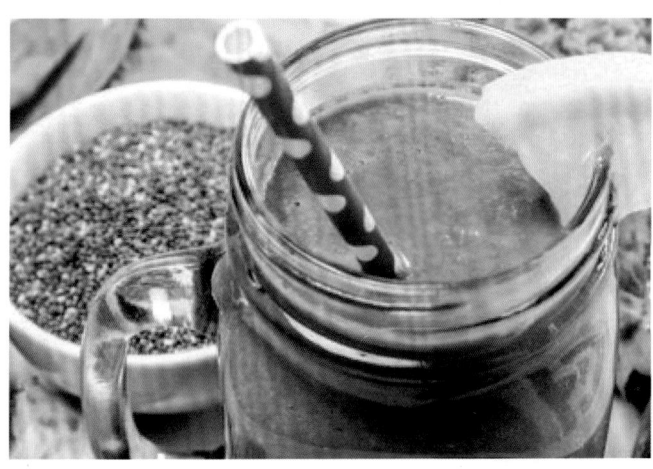

DAY 2 SMOOTHIE # 1
GREEN ISLAND DREAM

Key Vision Nutrients (per serving):

Lutein
Zeaxanthin
Vitamin C
Vitamin B12
Zinc

Ingredients:

- 2 cups fresh chopped kale
- ½ cup chopped broccoli
- 1 small banana
- 1 cup coconut water
- 2 tablespoons bee pollen
- ¼ cup dried goji berries

Prep Time: 30 seconds (plus overnight refrigeration)

Serves: 2

Steps:

1. Place all of the ingredients in the blender and refrigerate overnight.
2. In the morning, blend for 30 seconds.

Nutrition Data: 318 calories, 0.5g fat, 77.5g carbs, 14g protein, 14.2g fiber, 35.7g sugars, 173mg sodium

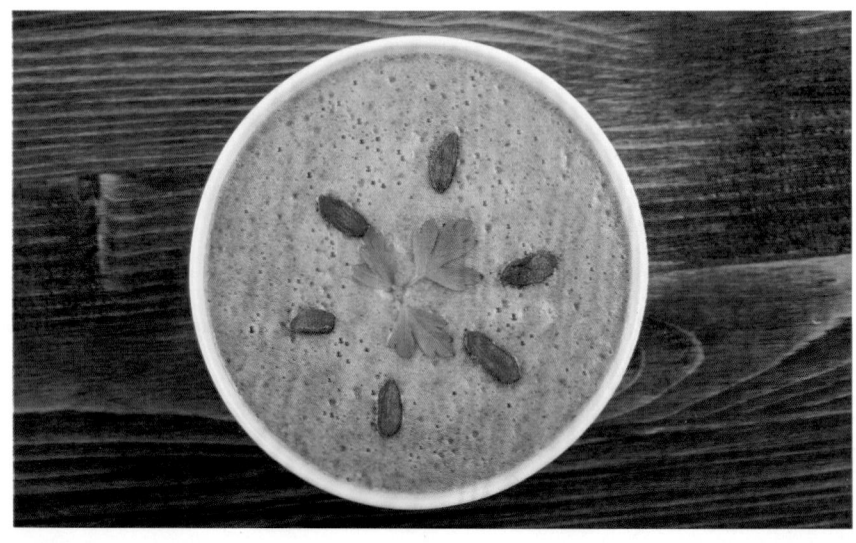

DAY 2 SMOOTHIE # 2
VEGGIE BOUQUET SMOOTHIE

Key Vision Nutrients (per serving):

Lutein

Zeaxanthin

Vitamin B12

Vitamin C

Zinc

Ingredients:

- 1 cup chopped cucumber
- 1 cup chopped spinach
- ¼ cup chopped tomatoes
- 2 tablespoons sliced green onion
- ½ cup chopped lettuce
- 1 tablespoon fresh chopped parsley
- 1 cup unsweetened almond milk

Prep Time: 50 seconds

Serves: 1

Steps:

1. Combine all of the ingredients in a blender.
2. Blend on high speed for 30 to 40 seconds until smooth, then serve with fresh parsley.

Nutrition Data: 80 calories, 3.9g fat, 10.6g carbs, 3.4g protein, 3.3g fiber, 3.6g sugars, 214mg sodium

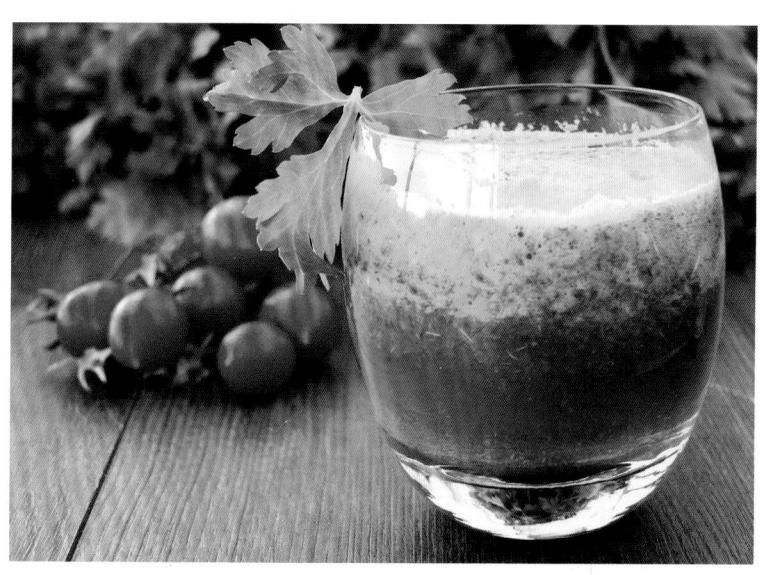

June 26, 2018

DAY 2 SMOOTHIE # 3 BLACKBERRY AND CRANBERRY SMOOTHIE

Key Vision Nutrients (per serving):

Lutein
Zeaxanthin
Vitamin B12
Vitamin B6
Zinc

Prep Time: 50 seconds

Serves: 1

Ingredients:

- ½ cup fresh blackberries
- ¼ cup coconut milk
- ¼ cup fresh cranberries
- 1 tablespoon egg white protein powder
- 1 tablespoon dark chocolate chips

Steps:

1. Combine the berries, coconut milk and protein powder in a blender.
2. Blend until smooth, about 30 to 40 seconds, then top with chocolate chips to serve.

Nutrition Data: 227 calories, 16.7g fat, 17.9g carbs, 4.5g protein, 6.1g fiber, 10.6g sugars, 36mg sodium

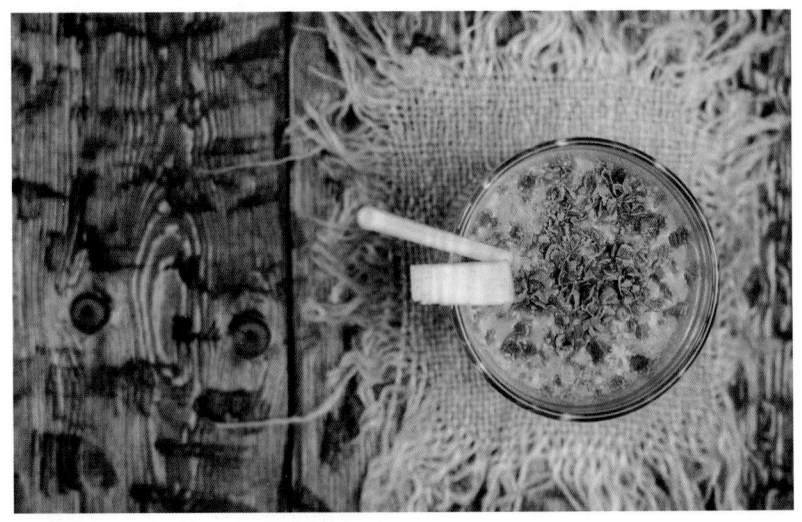

Jun 29, 2018

DAY 3 SMOOTHIE # 1
BILBERRY AND GRAPE SMOOTHIE

Key Vision Nutrients (per serving):

Lutein
Zeaxanthin
Vitamin B12
Vitamin B6
Zinc

Ingredients:

- ½ cup fresh or frozen bilberries
- ½ cup fresh grapes
- ¼ cup coconut milk
- 2 tablespoons fresh chopped mint
- Extra mint for garnish

Prep Time: 50 seconds

Serves: 1

Steps:

1. Combine the fruit, coconut milk, and chopped mint in a blender.
2. Blend for 30 to 45 seconds until smooth, then garnish with a fresh mint leaf.

Nutrition Data: 191 calories, 14.5g fat, 15.5g carbs, 2g protein, 3.1g fiber, 9.5g sugars, 13mg sodium

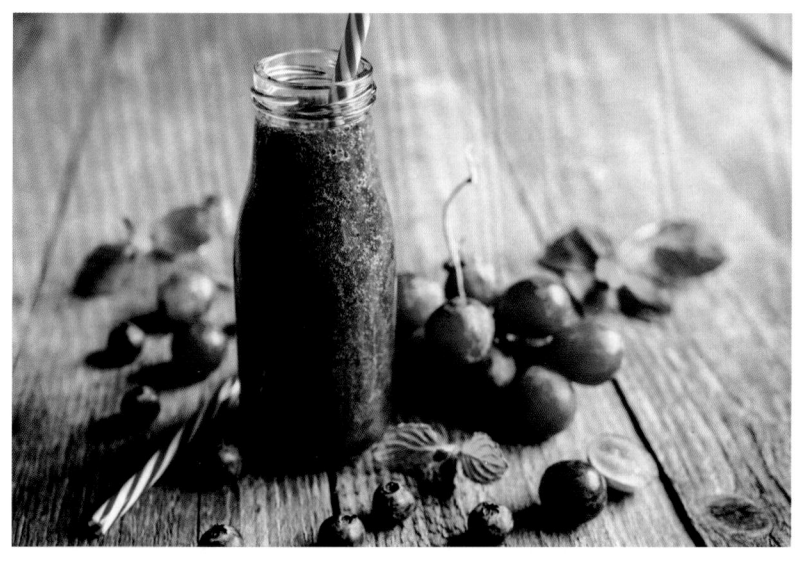

DAY 3 SMOOTHIE # 2
THE TOXIN TERMINATOR

Key Vision Nutrients (per serving):

Lutein
Zeaxanthin
Vitamin A
Vitamin C
Vitamin B12

Prep Time: 50 seconds

Serves: 2

Ingredients:

- 3 small apples, chopped
- 1 small stick of celery
- 1 cup chopped cucumber
- 1 cup chopped spinach
- 1 cup chopped kale
- 1 cup of ice

Steps:

1. Blend all ingredients together until smooth.

Nutrition Data: 203 calories, 0.7g fat, 52.4g carbs, 2.7g protein, 9.3g fiber, 35.8g sugars, 37mg sodium

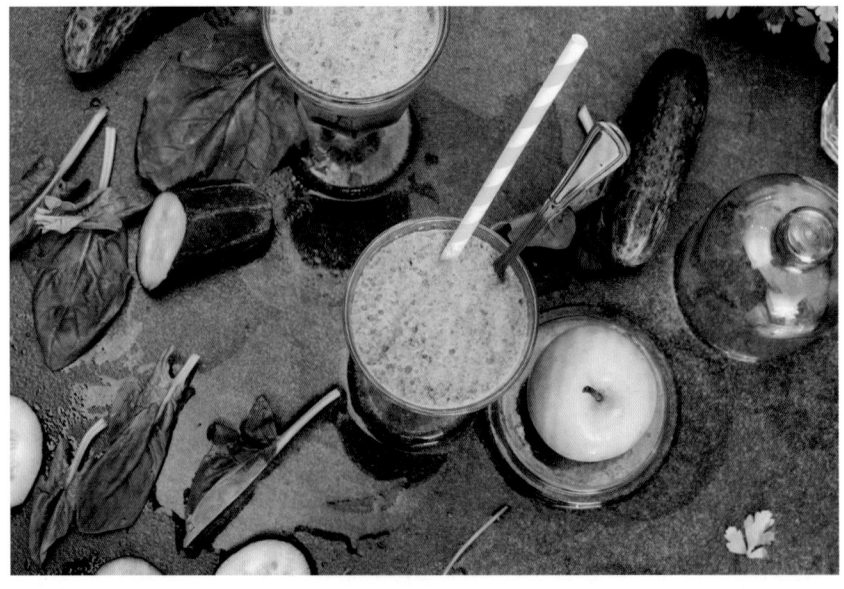

June 29, 2018

DAY 3 SMOOTHIE # 3
SUPER BERRY SMOOTHIE

Key Vision Nutrients (per serving):

Lutein

Zeaxanthin

Vitamin A

Vitamin B6

Vitamin C

Zinc

Ingredients:

- ½ cup frozen raspberries
- ½ cup frozen blueberries
- ½ cup tart cherry juice (unsweetened)
- ¼ cup water
- ¼ cup coconut milk
- ¼ cup raw almonds
- 1 teaspoon honey (optional)

Prep Time: 50 seconds

Serves: 2

Steps:

1. Combine the berries, cherry juice, and water in a blender and blend until smooth.
2. Add the coconut milk and almonds and blend. If desired, sweeten with the honey.
3. Divide between 2 glasses and serve, or store in the refrigerator for up to 4 days.

Nutrition Data: 245 calories, 13.4g fat, 31g carbs, 3.9g protein, 5g fiber, 23.3g sugars, 15mg sodium

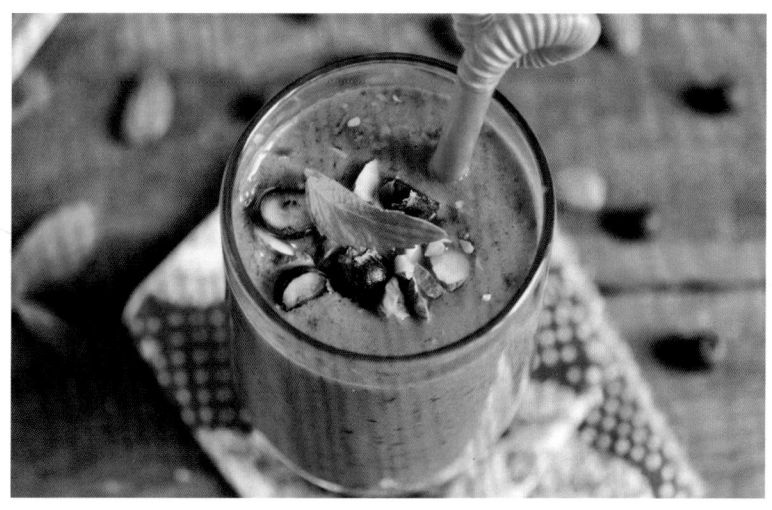

DAY 4 SMOOTHIE # 1
STRAWBERRY SPINACH POWER

Key Vision Nutrients (per serving):

Lutein

Zeaxanthin

Vitamin B12

Vitamin B16

Vitamin A

Vitamin C

Ingredients:

- 1½ cups coconut milk
- 5 strawberries, sliced
- ½ cup packed baby spinach
- 4 or 5 ice cubes

Prep Time: 50 seconds

Serves: 1

Steps:

1. Combine all of the ingredients in a blender and blend until smooth.
2. Divide between 2 glasses and serve, or store in the refrigerator for up to 4 days.

Nutrition Data: 90 calories, 6.2g fat, 8.2g carbs, 0.8g protein, 3g fiber, 3g sugars, 12mg sodium

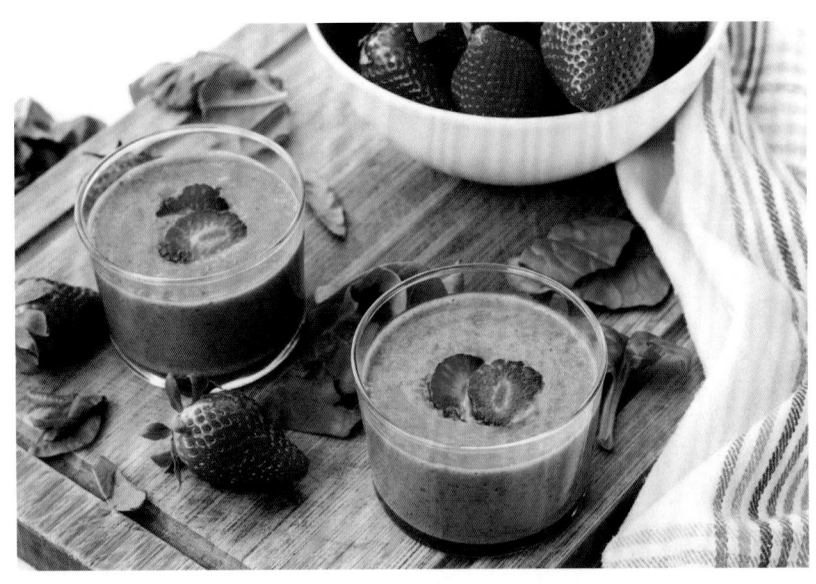

July 3, 2018

DAY 4 SMOOTHIE # 2 AVOCADO AND SPINACH SMOOTHIE

Key Vision Nutrients (per serving):

Lutein
Zeaxanthin
Omega-3
Vitamin C
Vitamin B12
Zinc

Ingredients:

- 2/3 cup chopped avocado
- 1 cup fresh chopped mango
- 2 tablespoons fresh lemon juice
- 1 tablespoon fresh grated ginger
- 1 cup chopped spinach
- 1 teaspoon honey
- 1 cup ice

Prep Time: 50 seconds

Serves: 2

Steps:

1. Combine the ingredients in a blender and blend until smooth.
2. Divide between 2 glasses and serve.

Nutrition Data: 176 calories, 10.1g fat, 22.2g carbs, 2.4g protein, 5.3g fiber, 14.9g sugars, 20mg sodium

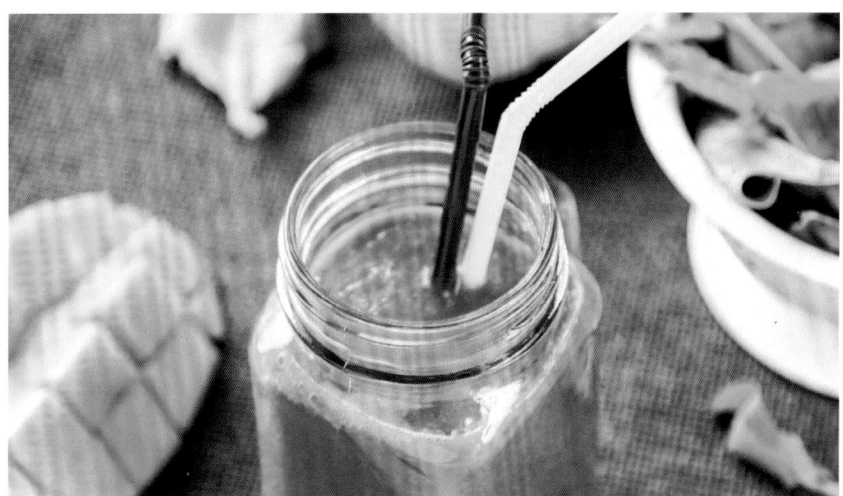

DAY 4 SMOOTHIE # 3
BLUEBERRY, PEACH AND
FLAXSEED SMOOTHIE

Key Vision Nutrients (per serving):

Lutein

Zeaxanthin

Omega-3

Vitamin B12

Vitamin B6

Vitamin C

Zinc

Ingredients:

- 1 small peach, pitted and chopped
- ¾ cup frozen blueberries
- ½ cup almond milk
- 2 tablespoons honey
- 1 tablespoon ground flaxseed
- 3 to 4 ice cubes

Prep Time: 50 seconds

Serves: 2

Steps:

1. Combine the ingredients in a blender and blend for 30 to 60 seconds, or until smooth.
2. Pour into glasses and serve immediately, or store in the refrigerator for up to 3 days.

Nutrition Data: 281 calories, 15.8g fat, 36.5g carbs, 3.2g protein, 4.8g fiber, 31.7g sugars, 11mg sodium

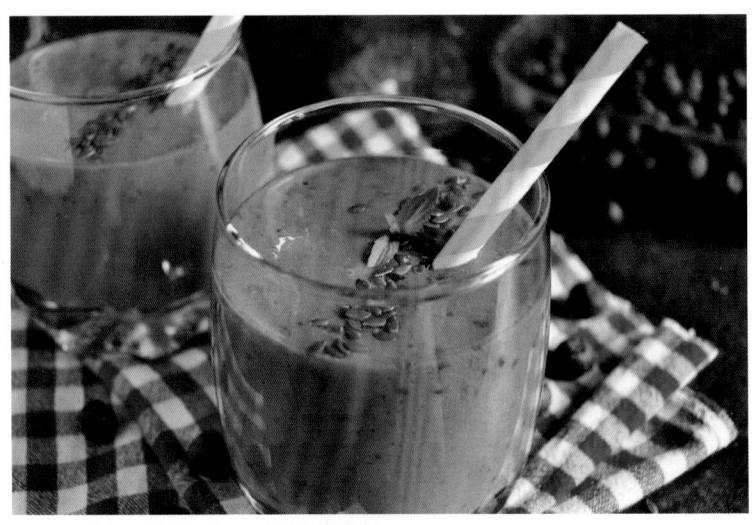

July 13, 2018

DAY 5 SMOOTHIE # 1
BERRY BEET SMOOTHIE

Key Vision Nutrients (per serving):

Lutein
Zeaxanthin
Vitamin C
Vitamin B12
Vitamin B6
Vitamin A

Ingredients:

- 1 cup coconut milk
- 1 cup sliced strawberries
- 1 small beet, peeled and chopped
- 1 cup blackcurrants
- 1 to 2 teaspoons agave nectar (optional)

Prep Time: 50 seconds

Serves: 2

Steps:

1. Combine the ingredients in a blender and blend for 30 to 60 seconds, or until smooth.
2. Pour into glasses and serve immediately, or store in the refrigerator for up to 3 days.

Nutrition Data: 371 calories, 29.2g fat, 29.8g carbs, 4.9g protein, 5.3g fiber, 15.3g sugars, 58mg sodium

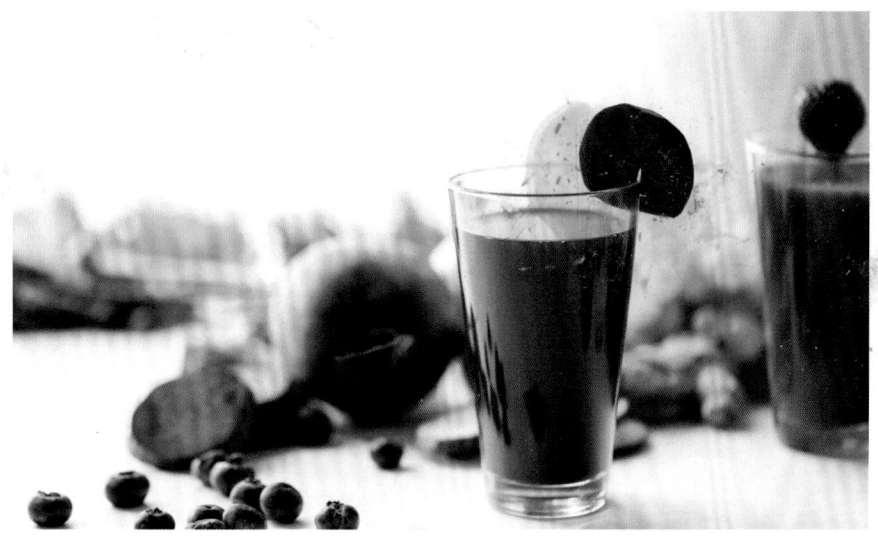

DAY 5 SMOOTHIE # 2
CLEAN BREEZE SMOOTHIE

Key Vision Nutrients (per serving):

Lutein
Zeaxanthin
Vitamin B12
Vitamin B6
Vitamin C
Zinc

Prep Time: 50 seconds

Serves: 2

Ingredients:

- 2 ripe and peeled kiwis
- ½ cup coconut milk
- 6 ice cubes
- 1 small cucumber, chopped
- 1 cup kombucha, ginger-flavored
- 1 cup chopped kale
- ½ cup cranberries
- Cilantro to taste

Steps:

1. Combine the ingredients in a blender and blend for 30 to 60 seconds, or until smooth.
2. Pour into glasses and serve immediately, or store in the refrigerator for up to 3 days.

Nutrition Data: 253 calories, 14.9g fat, 29.4g carbs, 4.2g protein, 5.9g fiber, 13.4g sugars, 34mg sodium

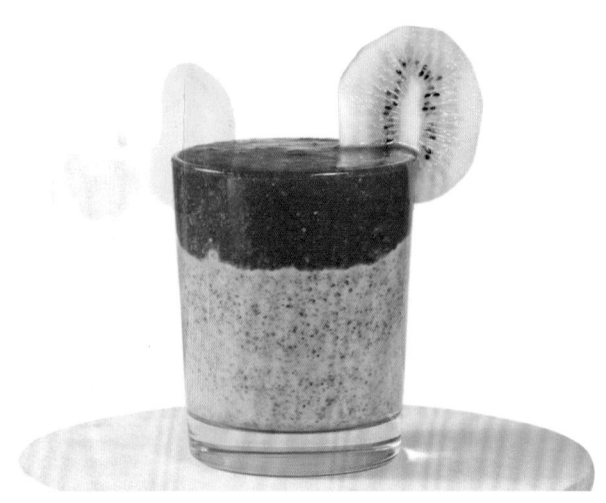

DAY 5 SMOOTHIE # 3 ANTIOXIDANT SMOOTHIE

Key Vision Nutrients (per serving):

Lutein

Zeaxanthin

Omega-3

Vitamin B6

Vitamin B12

Vitamin C

Zinc

Ingredients:

- 1 cup pomegranate juice, fresh and unsweetened
- 1 cup frozen blackberries
- 1 cup frozen dried goji berries
- 1 cup of water
- 1 tablespoon flaxseeds

Prep Time: 50 seconds

Serves: 2

Steps:

1. Combine the ingredients in a blender and blend for 30 to 60 seconds, or until smooth.
2. Pour into glasses and serve immediately, or store in the refrigerator for up to 3 days.

Nutrition Data: 319 calories, 4.3g fat, 67.3g carbs, 4g protein, 10.1g fiber, 55.6g sugars, 9mg sodium

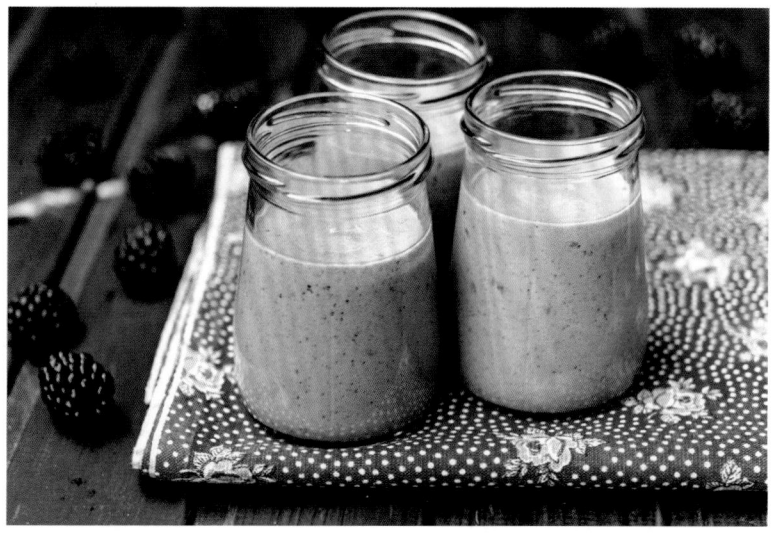

DAY 6 SMOOTHIE # 1
TROPICAL GRAPE SMOOTHIE

Key Vision Nutrients (per serving):

Lutein
Zeaxanthin
Vitamin B12
Vitamin B6
Vitamin C
Omega-3

Prep Time: 50 seconds

Serves: 1

Ingredients:

- 1½ cups frozen seedless red grapes
- 1 small frozen banana
- 1 cup sliced strawberries
- 1 teaspoon coconut cream concentrate
- 1 cup coconut water

Steps:

1. Place all ingredients in blender and blend on high speed until smooth.

Nutrition Data: 305 calories, 4.7g fat, 67.8g carbs, 5g protein, 9.8g fiber, 48.4g sugars, 259mg sodium

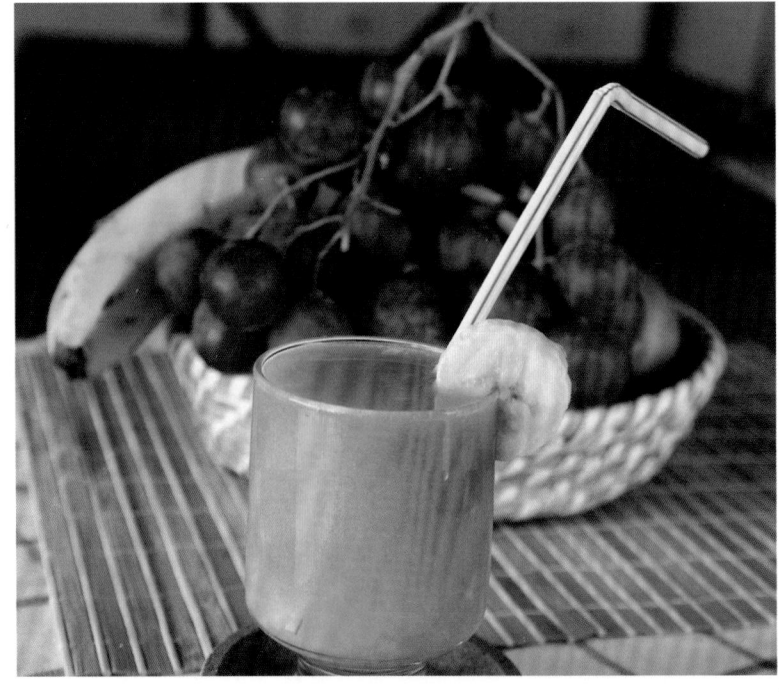

DAY 6 SMOOTHIE # 2
GREEN STRENGTH SMOOTHIE

Key Vision Nutrients (per serving):

Lutein

Zeaxanthin

Vitamin A

Vitamin C

Vitamin B12

Zinc

Prep Time: 50 seconds

Serves: 1

Ingredients:

- 1 small frozen banana
- 1/2 cup frozen strawberries
- 2 cups chopped spinach
- 1 cup organic unfiltered apple juice
- 1/2 cup coconut water
- 1 teaspoon spirulina powder

Steps:

1. Place all ingredients in blender and blend on high speed until smooth.

Nutrition Data: 263 calories, 1.3g fat, 63.2g carbs, 4.4g protein, 7.2g fiber, 43.3g sugars, 185mg sodium

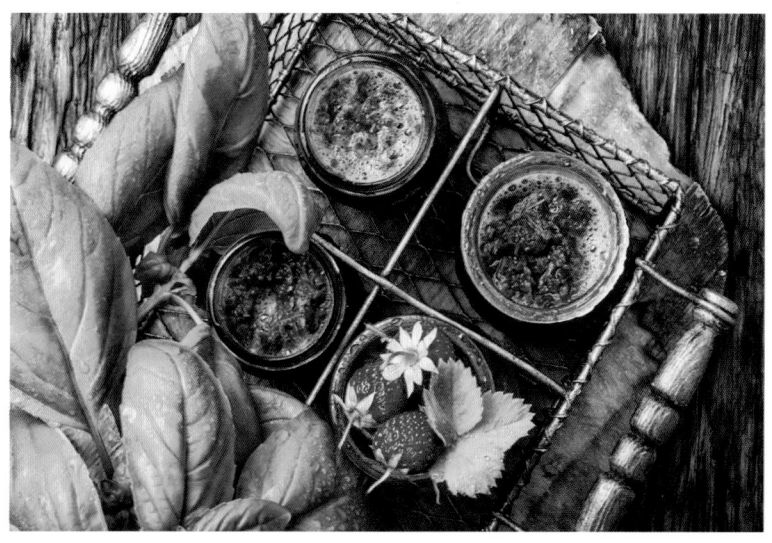

DAY 6 SMOOTHIE # 3 ORCHARD GREEN SMOOTHIE

Key Vision Nutrients (per serving):

Lutein
Zeaxanthin
Omega-3
Vitamin C
Vitamin B12
Vitamin B6
Zinc

Ingredients:

- 6 large carrots
- 1 cup frozen strawberries
- 2 seedless oranges, peeled
- 1/2 cup fresh chopped spinach
- 1/2 cup fresh chopped kale
- Juice from 1/2 lemon
- 1/4 teaspoon freshly grated ginger

Prep Time: 50 seconds

Serves: 2

Steps:

1. Feed the carrots through a juicer and collect the juice in a small container.
2. Add the carrot juice to a blender along with the rest of the ingredients.
3. Blend on high speed for 30 to 60 seconds, or until smooth.
4. Pour into glasses and serve immediately, or store in the refrigerator for up to 3 days.

Nutrition Data: 212 calories, 0.6g fat, 50.9g carbs, 4.8g protein, 11.7g fiber, 31.7g sugars, 166mg sodium

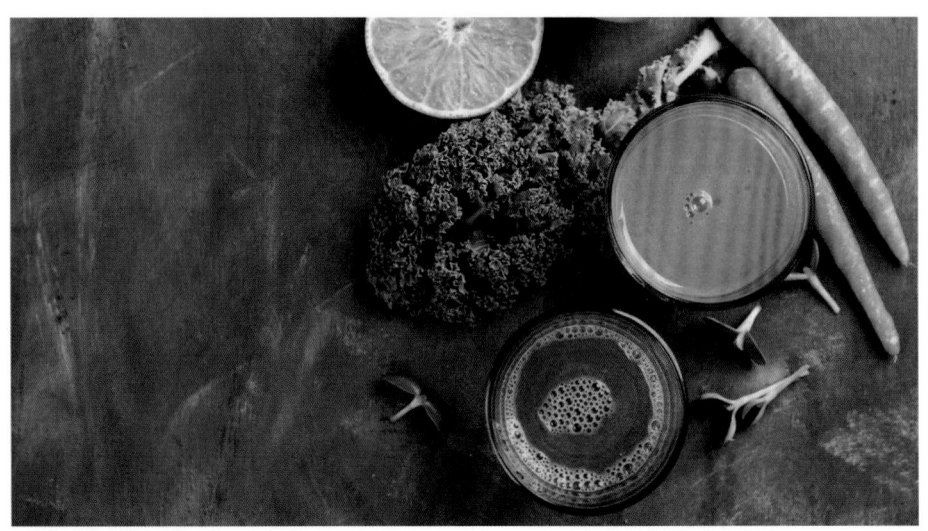

DAY 7 SMOOTHIE # 1
GREENS GALORE SMOOTHIE

Key Vision Nutrients (per serving):
Lutein
Zeaxanthin
Omega-3
Vitamin B12
Vitamin B6
Vitamin C
Zinc

Prep Time: 50 seconds

Serves: 2

Ingredients:

- 2 small frozen bananas
- 1 small green apple, cored
- 1 small pear, cored
- 1⁄2 cup fresh chopped spinach
- 1⁄2 cup fresh chopped kale
- 1⁄2 cup chopped romaine lettuce ✓
- 11⁄2 cups coconut water
- 1 tablespoon flaxseeds
- 1 teaspoon fresh lime juice ✓

Steps:

1. Place all ingredients in blender and blend on high speed until smooth.

Nutrition Data: 251 calories, 2.1g fat, 58.8g carbs, 4.3g protein, 10.8g fiber, 35.5g sugars, 206mg sodium

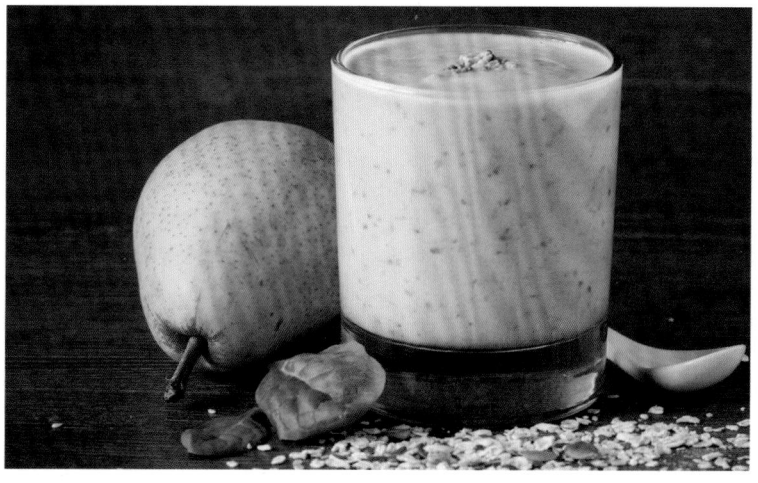

DAY 7 SMOOTHIE # 2
KALE POWER SMOOTHIE

Key Vision Nutrients (per serving):

Lutein
Zeaxanthin
Omega-3
Vitamin B12
Vitamin B6
Vitamin C
Zinc

Prep Time: 50 seconds

Serves: 2

Ingredients:

- 1 small frozen banana
- 1⁄2 cup frozen blackberries
- 2 cups fresh chopped kale
- 1 1⁄2 cups unsweetened almond milk
- 1 tablespoon raw honey
- 1⁄4 teaspoon ground cinnamon
- 1 tablespoon coconut oil

Steps:

1. Place all ingredients in blender and blend on high speed until smooth.

Nutrition Data: 215 calories, 9.8g fat, 32.4g carbs, 3.8g protein, 5.1g fiber, 16.6g sugars, 165mg sodium

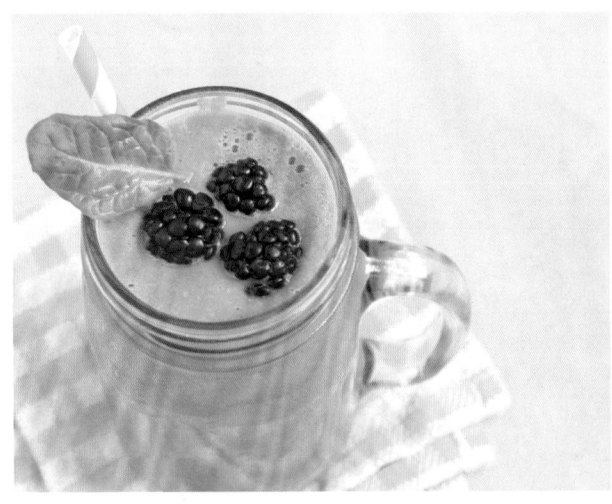

DAY 7 SMOOTHIE # 3
GREENS WITH A KICK SMOOTHIE

Key Vision Nutrients (per serving):

Lutein

Zeaxanthin

Omega-3

Vitamin B12

Vitamin B6

Vitamin C

Prep Time: 50 seconds

Serves: 2

Ingredients:

- 1½ cups frozen blueberries
- ½ cup chopped avocado
- 1 cup fresh chopped kale
- 1 cup coconut water
- 2 teaspoons raw honey
- 1 teaspoon cinnamon

Steps:

1. Place all ingredients in blender and blend on high speed until smooth.

Nutrition Data: 200 calories, 7.8g fat, 33.5g carbs, 3.5g protein, 7.5g fiber, 19.9g sugars, 144mg sodium

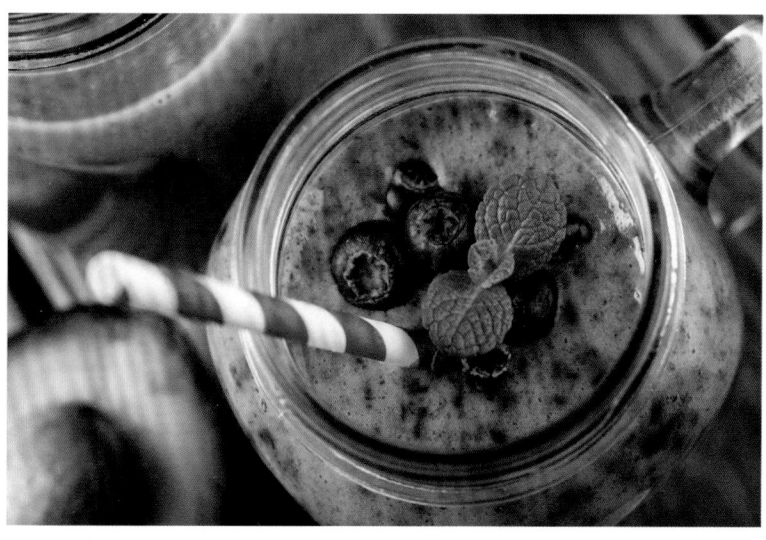

CHAPTER **FOURTEEN**

BRINGING IT ALL TOGETHER

In the previous 12 chapters, you have discovered everything you will ever need to know to reclaim your vision. I've shared with you everything I learned from Bunji in the Australian Outback, along with the modern world application that allowed my wife, and thousands of others, to attain 20/20 vision in just 21 days.

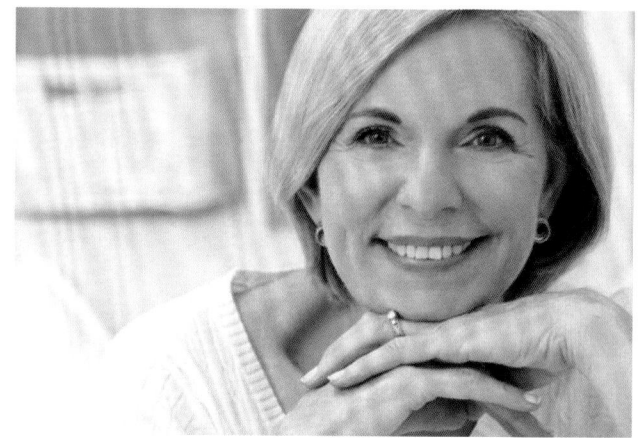

Simply add the smoothie protocol to your daily meals and you will start benefitting immediately from the awesome power of the antioxidants we have packed into each and every recipe.

Along this journey, you've discovered the things that don't work to improve your vision – and those that do – and this has freed you from the futility of eye exercises that don't produce results.

But it's also shown you the value of palming, something you should do on a daily basis. Aim to practice the six habits we covered in Chapter Six – they will allow you to maintain your vision as the years progress.

Thanks for taking this journey with me – I wish you a bright, clear future!

Chapter FIFTEEN

REFERENCES

(1)   https://www.ncbi.nlm.nih.gov/pubmed/20829643

(2)   https://nutritionreview.org/2013/04/vision-degenerative-disorders/

(3)   http://www.yelp.com/topic/oakland-problems-with-new-glasses

(4)   http://nyulangone.org/press-releases/contact-lens-wearers-take-note-your-eyes-may-get-more-infections-because-their-microbiomes-have-changed

(5)   https://www.optometry.unsw.edu.au/files/recruitment_poster_cvi_role_of_tear_lipids_final_ver1.pdf

(6)   https://www.optometry.unsw.edu.au/research/current-research

(7)   Liu, Z.; Pflugfelder, S. (January 2000). "The effects of long-term contact lens wear on corneal thickness, curvature, and surface regularity". Ophthalmology. **107** (1): 105–111. doi:10.1016/S0161-6420(99)00027-5. PMID 10647727.

(8)   Holden, B.A.; Sweeney, B.F.; Vannas, A.; Nilsson, K.T.; Efron, N. (November 1985). "Effects of long-term extended contact lens wear on the human cornea.". Invest. Ophthalmol. Vis. Sci. **26** (11): 1489–1501.

(9)   Holden, BA; Vannas, A; Nilsson, K; Efron, N; Sweeney, D; Kotow, M; La Hood, D; Guillon, M (June 1985). "Epithelial and endothelial effects from the extended wear of contact lenses.". Curr Eye Res. **4** (6): 739–42. doi:10.3109/02713688509017678.

(10)   Miller, D. (October 1968). "Contact Lens-Induced Corneal Curvature and Thickness Changes". Arch Ophthalmol. **80** (4): 430–432. doi:10.1001/archopht.1968.00980050432004.

(11)   Walline, J.; Jones, L.; Mutti, D.; Zadnik, K. (December 2004). "A Randomized Trial of the Effects of Rigid Contact Lenses on Myopia Progression". Arch Ophthalmol. **122**(12): 1760–1766. doi:10.1001/archopht.122.12.1760.

(12)   Millodot, M. (July 1978).

"Effect of Long-term Wear of Hard Contact Lenses on Corneal Sensitivity". Arch Ophthalmol. **96** (7): 1225–1227. doi:10.1001/archopht.1978.03910060059011. PMID 666631.

(13)   Patel, S.; McLaren, J.; Hodge, D.; Bourne, W. (April 2002). "Confocal Microscopy In Vivo in Corneas of Long-Term Contact Lens Wearers". Invest. Ophthalmol. Vis. Sci. **43** (4): 995–1003

(14)   http://www.allaboutvision.com/visionsurgery/lasik_complication_1.htm

(15)   https://www.gizmodo.com.au/2015/09/just-how-safe-is-laser-eye-surgery/

(16)   http://www.dailymail.co.uk/health/article-1334246/Tempted-laser-eye-surgery-Its-risks.html

(17)   http://www.cbsnews.com/news/lasik-eye-surgery-side-effects/

(18)   https://www.wddty.com/magazine/2016/march/the-new-dangers-of-laser-eye-surgery.html

(19)   https://www.ncbi.nlm.nih.gov/pubmed/19154276

(20)   Simon A and others. An evaluation of iridology. JAMA 242:13851387, 1979.

(21)   Knipschild P. Looking for gall bladder disease in the patient's iris. British Medical Journal 297:15781581, 1988.

(22)   http://www.abc.net.au/news/2015-04-08/prince-harry-may-struggle-to-keep-up-with-aboriginal-super-sight/6378066

(23)   http://www.aihw.gov.au/indigenous-observatory-eye-health/

(24)   https://nei.nih.gov/amd

(25)   https://www.ncbi.nlm.nih.gov/pmc/articles/PMC3705341/

(26)   Omega-3 long-chain polyunsaturated fatty acid intake and 12-year incidence of neovascular age-related macular degeneration and central geographic atrophy: AREDS report 30, a prospective cohort from the Age-Related Eye Disease Study. *American Journal of Clinical Nutrition.* December 2009.

(27)   Oily fish consumption, dietary docosahexaenoic acid and eicosapentaenoic acid intakes, and associations with neovascular age-related macular degeneration. *American Journal of Clinical Nutrition.* August 2008.

(28)   Essential n-3 fatty acids in pregnant women and early visual acuity maturation in term infants. *American Journal of Clinical Nutrition.* March 2008.

(29)   Topical Omega-3 and Omega-6 fatty acids for treatment of dry eye. *Archives of Ophthalmology.* February 2008.

(30)   Relation between dietary Omega-3 and Omega-6 fatty acids and clinically diagnosed dry eye syndrome in women. *American Journal of Clinical Nutrition.* October 2005.

(31)   Fish consumption, fish oil, Omega-3 fatty acids, and cardiovascular disease. American Heart Association Scientific Statement. *Circulation.* 2002.

(32)   Meta-analysis of dietary essential fatty acids and long-chain polyunsaturated fatty acids as they relate to visual resolution acuity in healthy preterm infants. *Pediatrics.* June 2000.

(33)   Dietary fat and fish intake and age-related maculopathy. *Archives of Ophthalmology.* March 2000.

(34)   NIH study provides clarity on supplements for protection against blinding eye disease. National Eye Institute

(35)   http://edition.cnn.com/2009/HEALTH/02/24/macular.degeneration.vitamins/index.html?iref=24hours

(36)   http://www.conference.net.au/chemeca2011/papers/437.pdf

(37)   http://www.abc.net.au/news/rural/2017-05-30/top-end-bush-tomato-plant-species-named-top-10/8568246

(38)   http://anfab.org.au/main.asp?_=Quandong

(39)   http://www.aihd.ku.edu/foods/Pigweed.html

(40)   http://www.bushfoodshop.com.au/wattleseed-ground/

(41)   https://www.survival.org.au/witchetty-grubs.php

(42)   http://www.sgm.com.au/html/nutrition.html

(43)   http://www.smh.com.au/entertainment/restaurants-and-bars/emu-the-other-red-meat-20111021-1mc04.html

(44)   https://www.scientificamerican.com/article/fact-or-fiction-carrots-improve-your-vision/

(45)   http://www.bushfoodshop.com.

au/bushfoodblog/finger-limes/

(46)   http://uk.blastingnews.com/health/2017/06/australias-native-bush-tucker-foods-001744427.html

(47)   http://anfab.org.au/main.asp?_=Muntries

(48)   http://www.bushfoodshop.com.au/riberries/

(49)   https://www.theguardian.com/lifeandstyle/australia-food-blog/2013/dec/11/bush-food-davidson-plums

(50)   https://www.aoa.org/patients-and-public/caring-for-your-vision/diet-and-nutrition/lutein?sso=y

(51)   Berendschot TT, Goldbohm RA, Klopping WA, van de Kraats J, van Norel J, van Norren D. Influence of Lutein supplementation on macular pigment, assessed with two objective techniques. Invest Ophthalmol Vis Sci 2007;41(11):3322-6.

(52)   Landrum JT, Bone RA, Joa H, Kilburn MD, Moore LL, Sprague KE. A one year study of the macular pigment: the effect of 140 days Lutein supplement. Exp Eye Res 1997;65(1):59-62.

(53)   http://www.abc.net.au/news/2015-04-08/prince-harry-may-struggle-to-keep-up-with-aboriginal-

super-sight/6378066

(54)   http://www.nutraingredients.com/Research/Long-term-lutein-intake-boosts-eyesight-in-cataract-patients

(55)   https://www.aoa.org/patients-and-public/caring-for-your-vision/diet-and-nutrition/lutein?sso=y

(56)   http://www.rnib.org.uk/eye-health-eye-conditions-age-related-macular-degeneration-amd/nutritional-supplements-age-related

(57)   http://www.ncbi.nlm.nih.gov/pmc/articles/PMC3705341/#B85-nutrients-05-01169

(58)   http://www.ncbi.nlm.nih.gov/pubmed/22005336

(59)   http://www.ncbi.nlm.nih.gov/pubmed/23645227

(60)   https://www.ncbi.nlm.nih.gov/pmc/articles/PMC3392472/

(61)   http://aoa.uberflip.com/i/239254-eye-health-nutrition-after-areds2

(62)   https://www.ncbi.nlm.nih.gov/pubmed/20829643

(63)   https://www.hoffmancenter.com/downloads/maculardegeneration.pdf

(64) http://macularhope.org/a-leading-cause-of-vision-loss/

(65) https://www.aoa.org/patients-and-public/caring-for-your-vision/diet-and-nutrition/lutein?sso=y

(66) Omega-3 long-chain polyunsaturated fatty acid intake and 12-year incidence of neovascular age-related macular degeneration and central geographic atrophy: AREDS report 30, a prospective cohort from the Age-Related Eye Disease Study. *American Journal of Clinical Nutrition.* December 2009.

(67) Oily fish consumption, dietary docosahexaenoic acid and eicosapentaenoic acid intakes, and associations with neovascular age-related macular degeneration. *American Journal of Clinical Nutrition.* August 2008.

(68) Essential n-3 fatty acids in pregnant women and early visual acuity maturation in term infants. *American Journal of Clinical Nutrition.* March 2009.

(69) Topical Omega-3 and Omega-6 fatty acids for treatment of dry eye. *Archives of Ophthalmology.* February 2014.

(70) Fish consumption, fish oil, Omega-3 fatty acids, and cardiovascular disease. American Heart Association Scientific Statement. *Circulation.* 2002.

(71) https://minnesota.aoa.org/documents/MN/Nutritional-Deficiencies-and-Ocular-Disease.pdf

(72) http://edition.cnn.com/2009/HEALTH/02/24/macular.degeneration.vitamins/index.html?iref=24hours

(73) https://www.ncbi.nlm.nih.gov/pubmed/16198909

(74) https://www.ncbi.nlm.nih.gov/pmc/articles/PMC2648137/

(75) C. I. Calero, E. Vickers, G. Moraga Cid, L. G. Aguayo, H. von Gersdorff, D. J. Calvo. **Allosteric Modulation of Retinal GABA Receptors by Ascorbic Acid**. *Journal of Neuroscience*, 2011; 31 (26): 9672 DOI: 10.1523/JNEUROSCI.5157-10.2011

(76) http://www.cbsnews.com/news/vitamin-c-may-help-protect-against-cataracts/

(77) https://www.ncbi.nlm.nih.gov/pubmed/17467747

(78) https://news.ohsu.edu/2011/07/14/ohsu-scientists-

discover-new-role-for-vitamin-c-in-the-eye-and-the-brain

(79) 2001). "A randomized, placebo-controlled, clinical trial of high-dose supplementation with vitamins C and E, beta carotene, and zinc for age-related macular degeneration and vision loss: AREDS report no. 8." *Arch Ophthalmol* 119(10): 1417-36.

(80) Chew, E. (2007). "Age-related eye disease study 2 protocol." National Eye Institute Protocol 07-EI-0025.

(81) http://www.bmj.com/content/352/bmj.i17

(82) http://www.naturalhealth365.com/blueberries.html/

(83) https://www.ncbi.nlm.nih.gov/books/NBK92756/

(84) http://www.ahchealthenews.com/2014/11/07/can-eating-grapes-improve-your-vision/http://ajcn.nutrition.org/content/66/4/1006S.short

(85) Nakaishi, H., Matsumoto, H., Tominaga, S., Hirayama, M. Effects of blackcurrant anthocyanoside intake on dark adaptation and VDT work induced transient refractive alteration in healthy humans. ALTERNATIVE MEDICINE REVIEW 2000, 5: 553-562

(86) Ikuyo Ohguroll, Hiroshi Ohgurol, Mitsuru Nakazawa Effects of anthocyanins in blackcurrant on retinal blood flow circulation of patients with normal tension glaucoma. A pilot study. HIROSAKI MEDICAL] OURNAL. 59: 23-32. 2007

(87) Hiroshi Ohguru, Ikuyo Ohguro, Maki Katai, Sachie Tanaka Two-year Randomized, Placebo Controlled Study of Blackcurrant Anthocyanins on Visual Field in Glaucoma. OPHTHALMOLOGICA 2012, 228:26-35

(88) https://www.ncbi.nlm.nih.gov/pubmed/22377796

(89) https://www.ncbi.nlm.nih.gov/pubmed/11483088?dopt=Abstract

(90) https://www.ncbi.nlm.nih.gov/pubmed/14662593?dopt=Abstract

(91) http://www.greenhealthwatch.com/newsstories/newsillnesses/bad-for-eyes.html

(92) http://blog.bostonsight.org/index.php/2013/12/the-impact-of-sugar-consumption-on-eye-health/

(93) https://www.rodalewellness.com/health/red-meat-and-blindness

(94) http://abcnews.go.com/GMA/story?id=126765&page=1

OUTBACK VISION PROTOCOL

HOME EYE TEST KIT

INSTRUCTION GUIDE

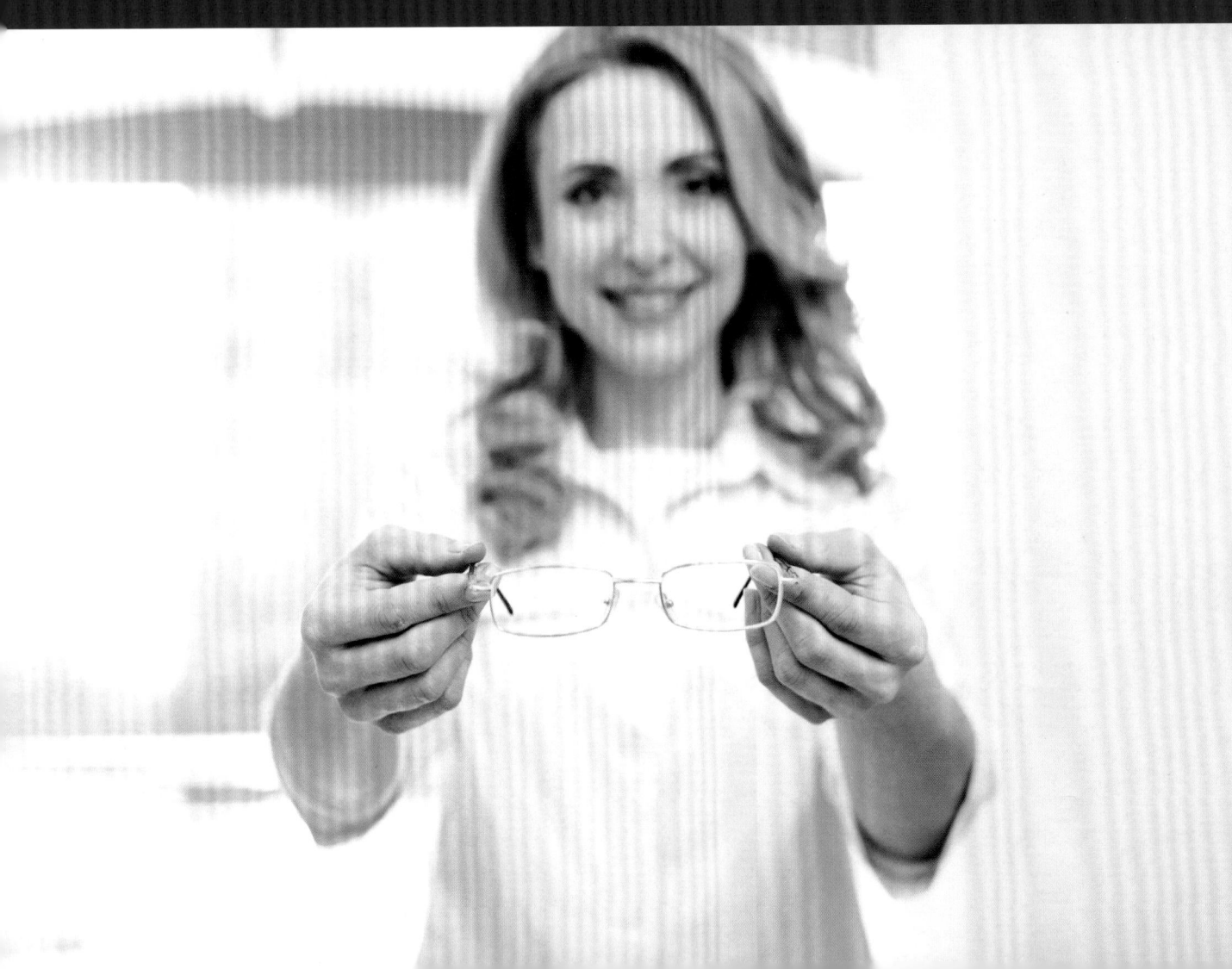

Introduction

The Outback Vision Protocol is designed to tackle the underlying cause of eye problems – free-radical damage. By boosting your intake of eight crucial antioxidants you can destroy free radicals and restore your vision permanently. Best of all? It's incredibly simple to do! All you have to do is follow the 7-day protocol, drinking three delicious smoothies per day, to harness the power of antioxidants to restore your vision. The longer you follow the protocol, the more pronounced your results are going to be, so don't give up!

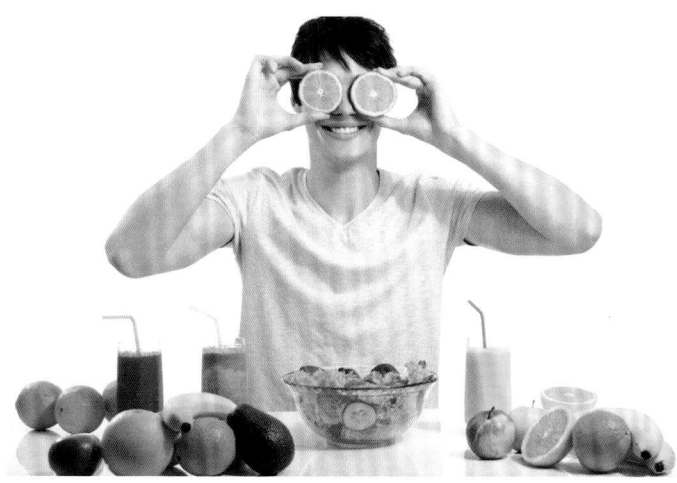

Every person's body is different and you may be starting in a different place than someone else. The Outback Vision Protocol is guaranteed to restore your vision but, depending on your current prescription, it might take a little longer for some people than for others. It is important that you stick to the protocol, however, and don't lose hope! It will take some time for your body to heal from all of that free-radical damage and for your eyes to be restored to healthy vision.

What can you do in the meantime while all of those antioxidants are doing their job? You can use this at home eye test kit to monitor your progress! This at-home test consists of twelve different charts and tests as well as detailed instructions for their use.

Why is Regular Testing Important?

If you are starting the Outback Vision Protocol with a low prescription, you may notice results in as few as 7 days. For higher prescriptions, however, the healing and restoration process may take a little longer. Rather than just sitting around waiting for your vision to become perfectly clear, take the time to test your vision at least once a week as you complete the protocol. Testing your vision regularly will help you to monitor the results and when you see the protocol doing what it is supposed to do, you'll be that much more motivated to keep going!

In addition to performing these at-home vision tests to monitor the progress of your Outback Vision Protocol, you should still see your ophthalmologist on a regular basis – at least once a year. While these tests may help you monitor the strength of your vision, only an ophthalmologist can diagnose eye problems. If you continue to experience pain, double vision, dark spots, or halos in your vision after completing the protocol, you may want to schedule an appointment with your eye doctor.

As you prepare to take your at-home eye tests, there are a few things you should do in preparation. First, start with 30 seconds of palming to rest your eyes and calm your mind. Sit at the table in a comfortable chair and use pillows or cushions to rest your elbows on so that your hands are at eye level. Close your eyes and cover both eyes with your hands, slightly cupping them so you aren't touching your eyes. Your fingers can be interlaced and rested on your forehead. Adjust your hands until no light gets through then close your eyes and breathe slowly for at least 30 seconds.

Once you have finished palming, start with the first eye test exercise. Try to remain calm and focused throughout the testing period so that you'll have clear results. You may find it helpful to jot down some notes for each test so you can track your progress. Throughout the course of the testing period, take short breaks to breathe, blink, and adjust your posture so you remain relaxed. You can also take a break or two for palming if your eyes start to become strained or sore.

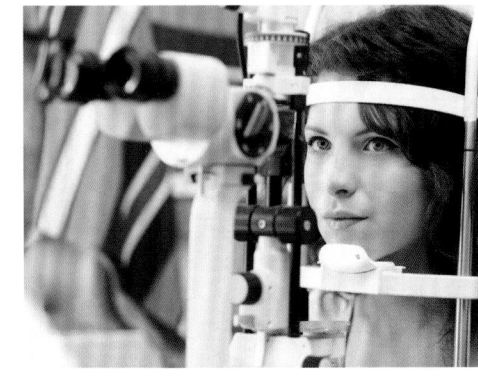

At-Home Eye Tests

Included in this home eye test kit is an assortment of different tests you can use to check your vision. Each of these tests will give you insight into how much your vision is improving as you work your way through the Outback Vision Protocol. Keep in mind that these tests are for your own use and their sole purpose is to gauge your progress – they are not a substitute for your annual eye exam and they cannot be used to detect or diagnose any vision problems. Feel free to perform the tests in the order listed or pick and choose from the list. If you consistently

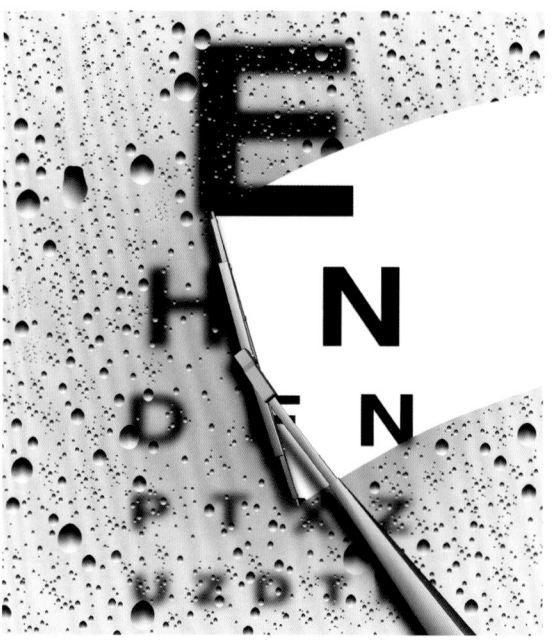

perform well in one or more of the tests, you can skip those the next time and focus on the other tests until you are able to complete each test with the highest degree of accuracy.

Before you get started with the home eye test kit, take a moment to familiarize yourself with the type of tests you'll be performing. Here is a quick overview of the eye tests involved in this kit:

1 Basic Eye Chart – This is the same eye test you take when you see your optometrist – it consists of different letters at different sizes and you must identify them to test your vision.

2 Visual Acuity Test – Also known as the "E Game," this test measures your distance visual acuity. It consists of multiple letter "E"s in different sizes and orientations – you must identify the direction of each letter "E."

3 Astigmatism Test – This test will help you to test whether you have astigmatism or not by determining whether some of the lines in different shapes are darker or thicker than others.

4 **Near Vision Test 1** – This test consists of four lines of text at different sizes to determine the strength of your near vision.

5 **Near Vision Test 2** – This test consists of four black circles of two different sizes juxtaposed over a green or red background to test your near vision.

6 **Color Vision** – This test consists of colored circles with colored numbers inside and it is designed to test your color vision.

7 **Amsler Grid Test** – This test is designed to detect macular degeneration – it consists of a large grid with many small squares and a dot in the middle.

8 **Contrast Vision Test** – This test consists of block letters in different sizes, fading from solid black to very light gray and it is designed to test your contrast vision.

9 **Reading Strength Test** – The purpose of this test is to have a clear measure of the strength of your near vision so you can more accurately monitor your progress.

10 **Convergence Test** - This test is designed to test your convergence skills, or how well your eyes work together.

11 **Fusion Test** - This test is designed to measure and strengthen your fusion skills, or the ability of your left and right eyes to fuse two images together.

12 **Divergence Test** - This test is designed to measure and strengthen your divergence skills – your ability to maintain a single central image while viewing images on either side as well.

Detailed Instructions
for At Home Eye Tests

1 Basic Eye Chart

This is the type of eye test you normally perform at the eye doctor. It is designed to test your vision and it will give you an idea as to the overall strength of your vision on a scale from 20/200 to 20/20 with 20/20 being perfect vision.

Preparation:

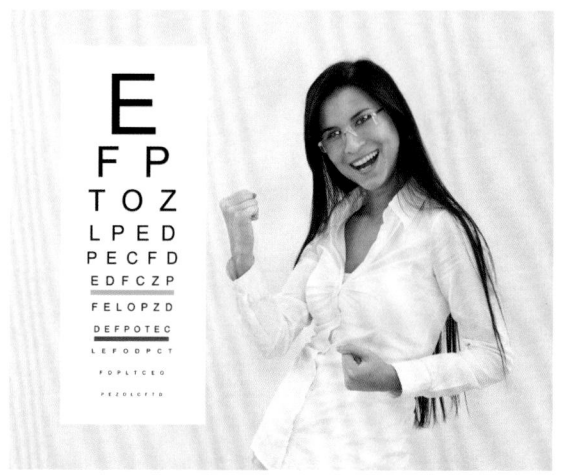

1. Hang the chart on the wall in a well-lit area.

2. Stand a distance of 10 feet away from the chart when performing the test.

Performing the Test:

1. Carefully cover your left eye and look at the chart.

2. Read the top line of letters then keep moving down until you can no longer clearly identify the letters.

3. Repeat the test covering your right eye.

4. Have someone record your responses to the test then compare them to the chart.

Test Results:

As indicated on the chart itself, being able to read the bottom line clearly indicates 20/20 vision. If you can only read the top line clearly, you have 20/200 vision – the stronger your vision, the lower the second number.

② Visual Acuity Test

This test is designed to assess your visual acuity by identifying the direction of the opening in letter "E"s of different size. The more clearly you are able to identify the direction of the opening for smaller and smaller "E"s, the stronger your vision.

Preparation:

1 Adjust the size of the chart until the bar printed at the bottom measures 100mm.

2 Hang the chart on the wall in a well-lit area.

3 Stand a distance of 10 feet away from the chart when performing the test.

Performing the Test:

1 Carefully cover your left eye and stand 10 feet away from the chart.

2 Have someone cover the chart, illuminating just one "E" at a time.

3 Identify the direction in which the open end of the "E" is pointed each time, working your way down the chart.

4 Repeat the test while covering your right eye, working your way down the chart.

5 Have someone record your responses to the test then compare them to the chart.

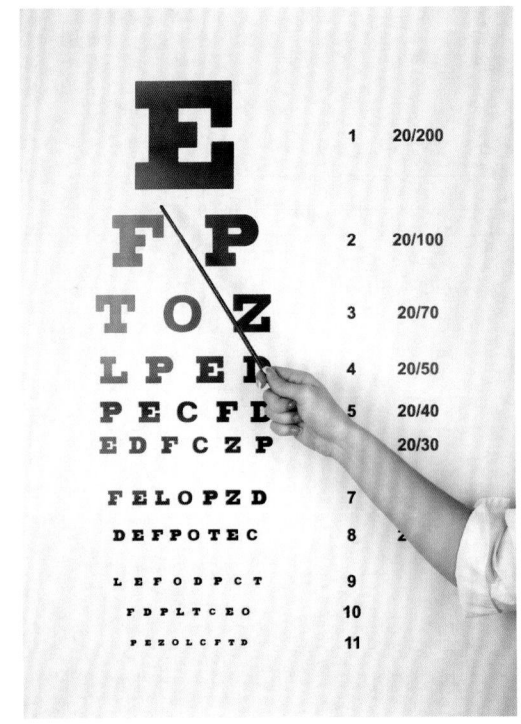

Test Results:

Use the chart to determine the strength of your visual acuity. If you are able to identify the bottom line accurately it indicates 20/20 or perfect vision. If you can only read the top line clearly, you have 20/200 vision – the stronger your vision, the lower the second number.

3 Astigmatism Test

Astigmatism is a condition caused by irregular curvature of the lens or cornea and it typically causes blurred vision in one or both eyes. Because astigmatism can affect one or both eyes, you'll need to perform this test on each eye individually. Simply look at the image and determine whether any of the lines look darker or bolder than the rest.

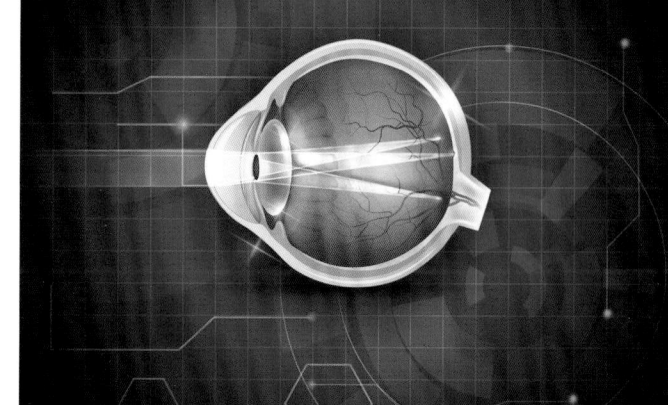

Preparation:

1 Hang the chart on the wall in a well-lit area.

2 Stand a distance of 2 to 3 meters away from the chart when performing the test.

Performing the Test:

1 Carefully cover your left eye then look at the top image – do all of the lines appear to have the same thickness and clarity?

2 Keep your left eye covered then focus on the second image – do all of the lines seem equally clear and dark?

3 Keep your left eye covered and focus on the third image – are all of the heavy lines radiating out from the center equal in thickness and intensity?

4 Cover your right eye and repeat the three tests.

Test Results:

If you have astigmatism, some of the black lines may appear thicker than others or they might appear to be distorted. If all of the lines seem equal in thickness and boldness, you probably don't have astigmatism.

4 Near Vision Test 1

This test is designed to check your near vision - simply hold or hang the test 40 cm away from your eyes. The more of the text you can read, the stronger your near vision.

Preparation:

1 Print the test on thick paper.

2 Hold the test 40 cm from your eyes or hang it on a wall and stand 40 cm away.

Performing the Test:

1 Look at the text printed on the sheet of paper.

2 Read the text as far down as you are able to do so clearly then compare your results.

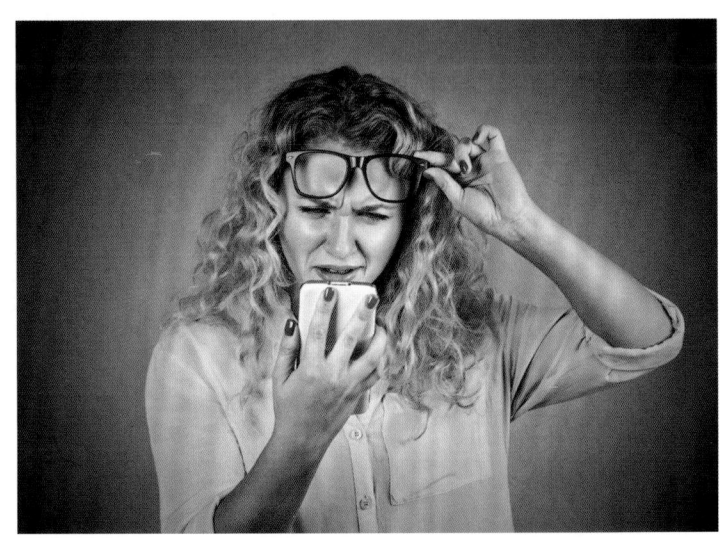

Test Results:

After reading the test, compare your response to the print on the test – how many words did you accurately read and how far down could you go? The more accurately you are able to read the text down to the bottom line, the stronger your near vision.

5 Near Vision Test 2

This test is designed to check your near vision to determine whether you are myopic, presbyopic, or have perfect near vision. Simply hold or hang the test 40 cm away from your eyes.

Preparation:

1 Print the test on thick paper.

2 Hold the test 40 cm from your eyes or hang it on a wall and stand 40 cm away.

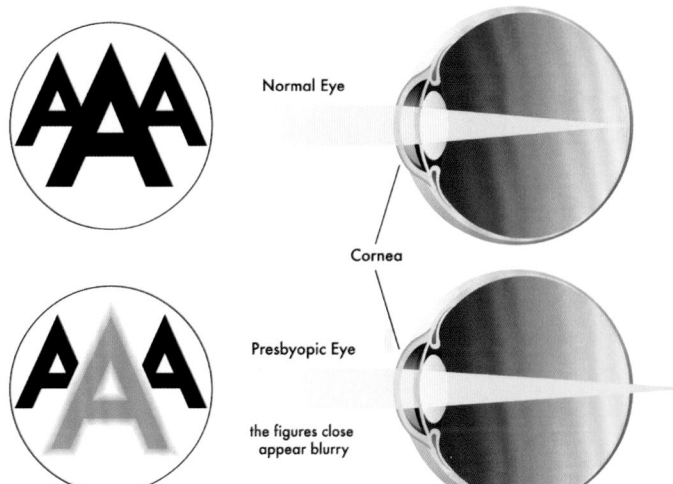

Performing the Test:

1 Look at the black rings printed on the green background on the left side of the test.

2 Look at the black rings printed on the red background on the right side of the test.

3 Ask yourself whether the rings seem darker on the left side or the right side, or if they are equally dark on both sides.

Test Results:

If the circles on the either background seem darker you could be myopic – this means that your near vision is too strong. If the circles appear equally dark on both sides you have strong near vision.

⑥ Color Vision

Color blindness tends to affect men more than women and there are different degrees of color blindness. This test consists of colored circles with colored numbers hidden within. If you are able to correctly identify all of the numbers you do not have color blindness.

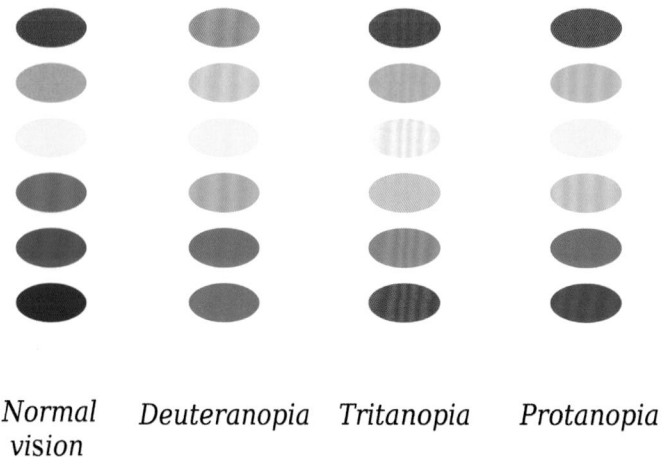

Normal vision Deuteranopia Tritanopia Protanopia

Preparation:

1 Print the test in full color and hold it in front of you – the distance does not matter.

Performing the Test:

1 Cover your left eye and view the chart in front of you.

2 Identify the number hidden in the circle on the top left of the chart.

3 Work your way through the chart until you've identified all ten numbers.

4 Repeat the test with your right eye covered.

Test Results:

Compare your results to the answers. If you are able to identify all of the numbers correctly, there are no problems with your color vision.

7 Amsler Grid Test

This test is designed to monitor the function of your macula which is the central area of your vision. Macular degeneration and other disorders can cause distortion of the retina which may change your vision. The Amsler Grid test is designed to detect macular degeneration.

Preparation:

1 Print the grid on thick paper and adjust the size as needed so it measures 4-by-4 inches.

2 Hang the grid on the wall in a well-lit area and stand 14 inches away.

Performing the Test:

1 Carefully cover your left eye and look at the grid, focusing on the dot in the center.

2 View the horizontal and vertical lines of the grid with your peripheral vision – do they appear distorted or broken?

3 Repeat the test with your right eye covered.

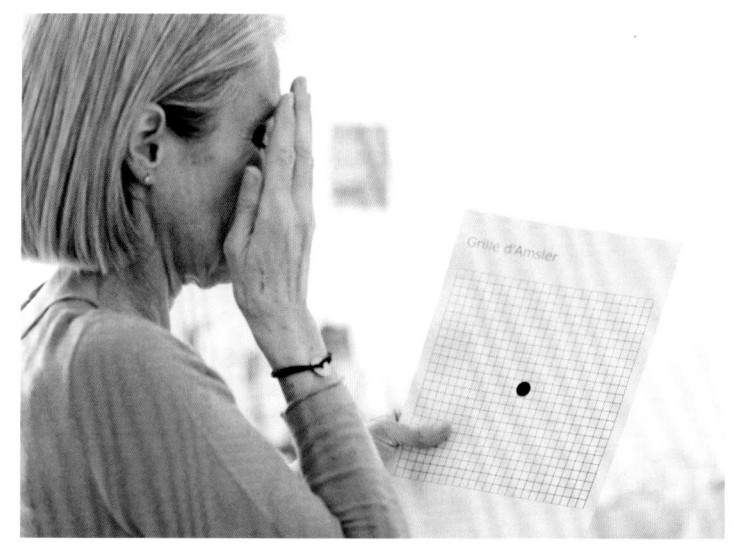

Test Results:

When performing this test with perfect vision, none of the lines on the grid should be broken or distorted – they should meet at all crossing points with no spaces.

8 Contrast Vision Test

Though the contrast vision test may not seem as important as the others, your contrast vision is still an indication of eye health. If you have a problem with your contrast vision, it could cause your eyes to become fatigued more quickly and that can lead to problems. Changes in your contrast vision may signify a problem with your eye health such as developing glaucoma.

Preparation:

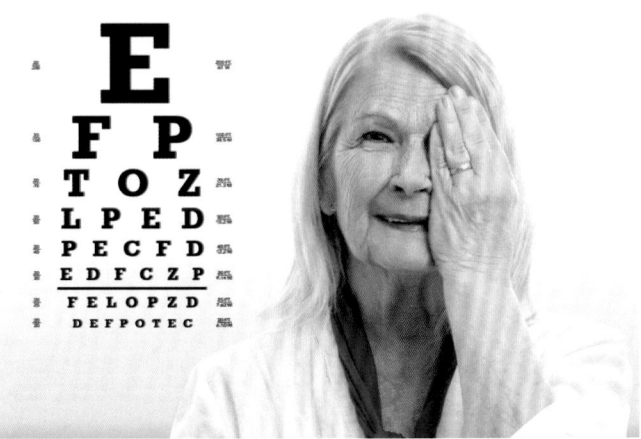

1. Hang the chart on the wall in a well-lit area.

2. Stand a distance of 40 cm away from the chart when performing the test.

Performing the Test:

1. Carefully cover your left eye and look at the chart.

2. Read the letters on the chart from left to right, starting at the top of the chart.

3. Continue reading the letters until you are no longer able to make them out then compare your results to the answer sheet.

4. Cover your right eye and repeat the test, reading the letters and recording your answers.

Test Results:

This test is known as the Mars Letter Contrast Sensitivity Test and each letter is correlated with a certain value. For your purposes with the Outback Vision Protocol, however, you simply want to make note of how far down the chart you are able to clearly identify the letters. As your vision improves, you should eventually be able to make it all the way through.

⑨ Reading Strength Test

This test is designed to test the strength of your reading vision, another aspect of your near vision. The purpose of this test is to have a clear measure of the strength of your near vision so you can more accurately monitor your progress while you complete the Outback Vision Protocol.

Preparation:

1 Print the chart in full, adjusting the size so it measures 5 inches wide.

2 Hold the chart level at comfortable reading distance in front of your face, about 14 inches.

Performing the Test:

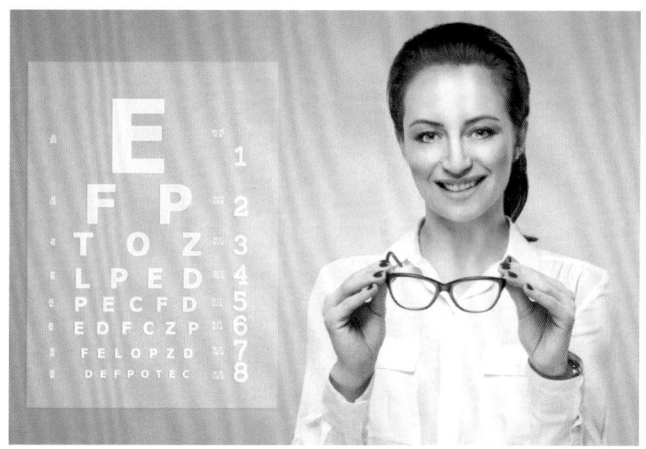

1 Start with the bottom line and see if you are able to read it clearly.

2 If you are able to read the bottom line, work your way up until the text is no longer clear.

Test Results:

As you work your way up the chart, take note of the highest line you can read clearly then compare your results to the number on the chart. Make note of this number and compare it to your results the next time you complete the test.

🔟 Convergence Test

This test is designed to test your convergence skills, or how well your eyes work together. By focusing on a point halfway between your eyes and the text you create a 3D effect similar to the way you view the Magic Eye pictures to see a 3D image.

Preparation:

1 Print the chart in full and hold it at arm's length.

2 Extend the index finger of your other hand and hold it in the center of your vision halfway between your eyes and the chart.

Performing the Test:

1 Focus on the tip of your finger.

2 In the background, you should see a column of text doubled behind the two printed columns – this makes the image look 3D.

3 Read the text in the 3D column, moving as slowly as you need to, working your way down the chart.

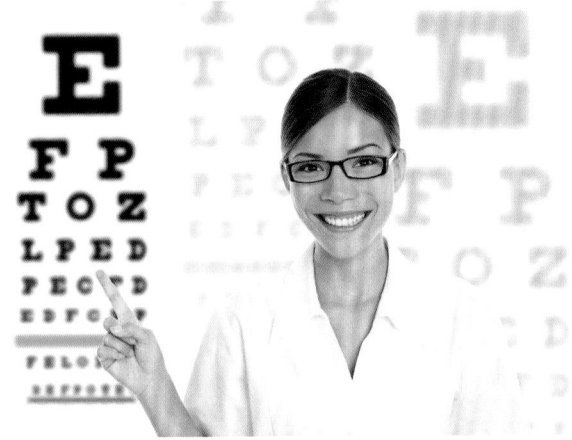

Test Results:

The first few times you try this exercise you may not have great results but you'll get better as you go. The stronger your vision becomes and the more your eyes learn to work together, the better you will become at convergence and you'll eventually make it through the entire chart.

⑪ Fusion Test

This test is designed to measure and strengthen your fusion skills, or the ability of your left and right eyes to fuse two images together. Your eyes do this automatically when you read but it can take some practice to use the skill on demand.

Preparation:

① Print the chart in full and hold it in front of your face so the paper touches your nose.

Performing the Test:

① Focus on the space between the two circles, fusing them together into a third circle.

② Slowly move the chart further away from your face while keeping the circles fused.

③ If the circles start to separate, stop and correct yourself before moving forward.

④ Keep going until you are able to maintain fusion with the chart at arm's length.

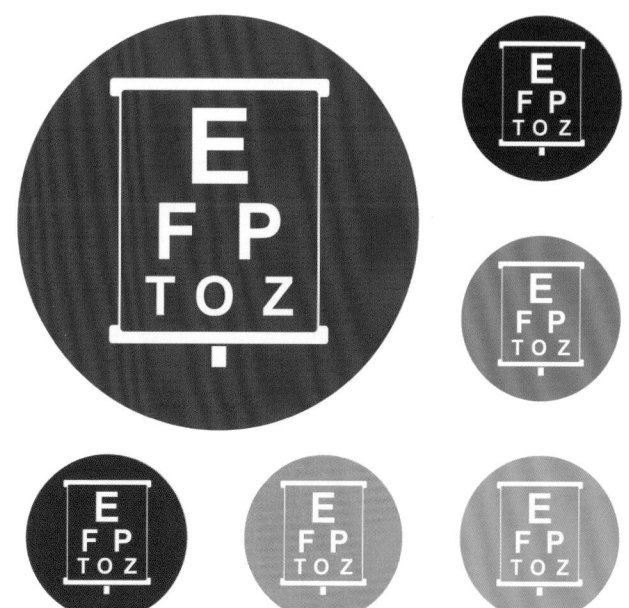

Test Results:

Working slowly, you should be able to develop your fusion skills as you move the paper further from your face. The ultimate test is, once the chart is at arm's length, looking away and then being able to instantly see three perfect circles when you look back at the chart. Keep in mind that this may take several tries to master as your vision becomes stronger.

12 Divergence Test

In ophthalmological terms, divergence is the simultaneous outward movement of both eyes away from each other, generally in an effort to maintain binocular vision. This test is designed to measure and strengthen your divergence skills – your ability to maintain a single central image while viewing images on either side as well.

Preparation:

1 Print the chart in full and hold it in front of your face so the paper touches your nose.

2 Align the chart so there is one cross below each eye.

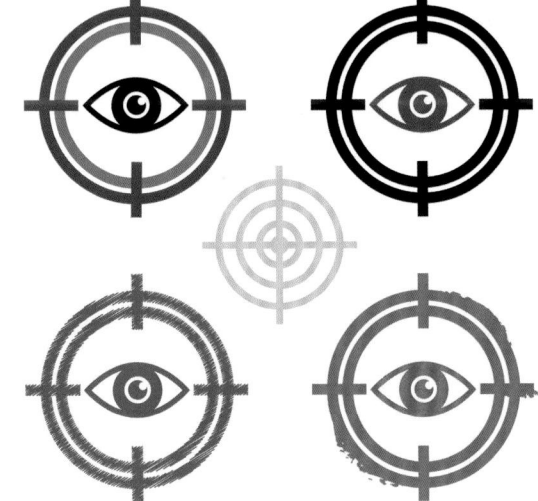

Performing the Test:

1 Look at an object in the distance then slowly bring the chart up to block your view – there should be one cross directly in front of each eye.

2 Continue to focus your eyes as if looking at that distant object – don't look at the crosses.

3 Notice the crosses in front of your eyes without focusing on them until you see one large, blurry cross.

4 Take a breath and blink your eyes while keeping the large cross in your vision.

5 Slowly move the chart away from your face until you see two crosses on either side of the large cross at a distance of 2 or 3 inches.

6 Keep all three crosses in your vision as you move the chart further away – if you lose the crosses at any point, move it back until you have them again.

7 Keep working until you can maintain three crosses in your vision at any distance.

Test Results:

This test takes a lot of practice to master, so work slowly. Once you are able to maintain the large central cross at a distance of two or three inches, work slowly to maintain it at larger distances. When you lose the central cross, bring the chart back to your nose and start again.

Basic Eye Chart

20/200	C S	1
20/100	D V O H	2
20/80	O H V C K	3
20/63	H Z C K O	4
20/50	N C K H D	5
20/40	D H O S Z	6
20/32	V R N D O	7
20/25	C Z H K S	8
20/20	O R Z S K	9

Visual Acuity Test
(Read in good light at 10 feet)

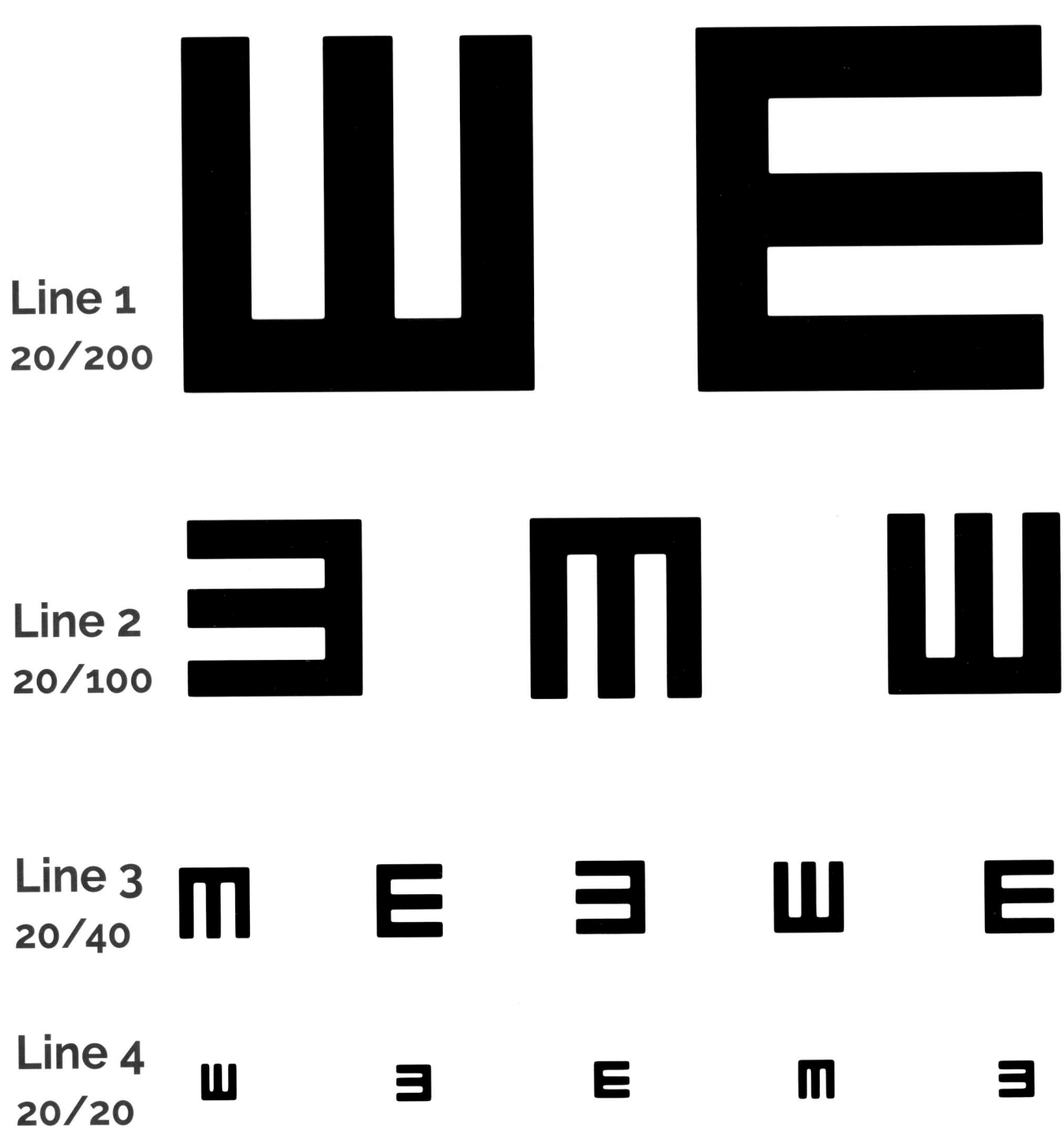

Line 1
20/200

Line 2
20/100

Line 3
20/40

Line 4
20/20

100 Milimeter Calibration Bar
(If not 100 mm, see text of visual acuity page)

Astigmatism Test

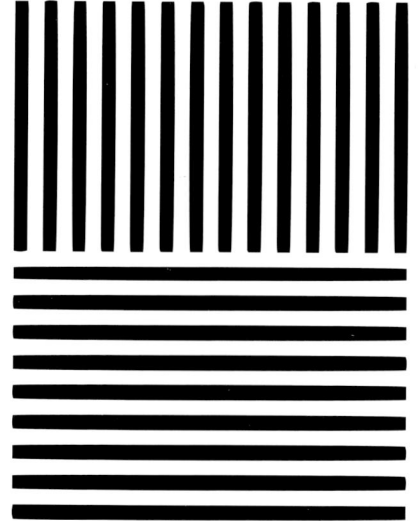

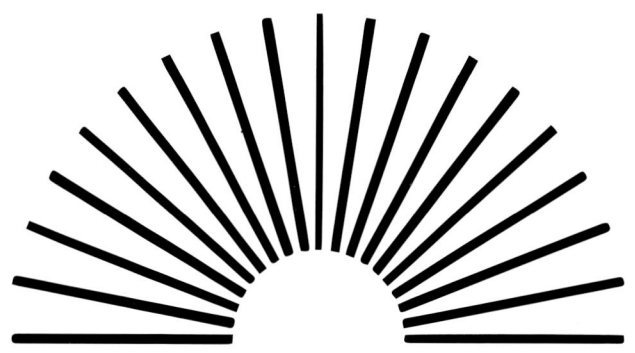

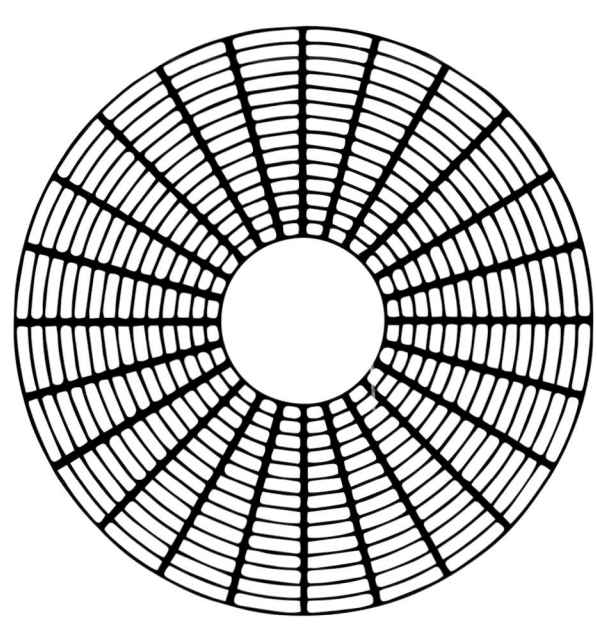

Near Vision Test

Near Vision Test 1

Being able to see well at any distance, without the need to constantly

fiddle his glasses, is increasingly necessary when one's eyes are tired.

With progressives lenses all presbyopes can still have most

of the visual acuity that they always had

Near Vision Test 2

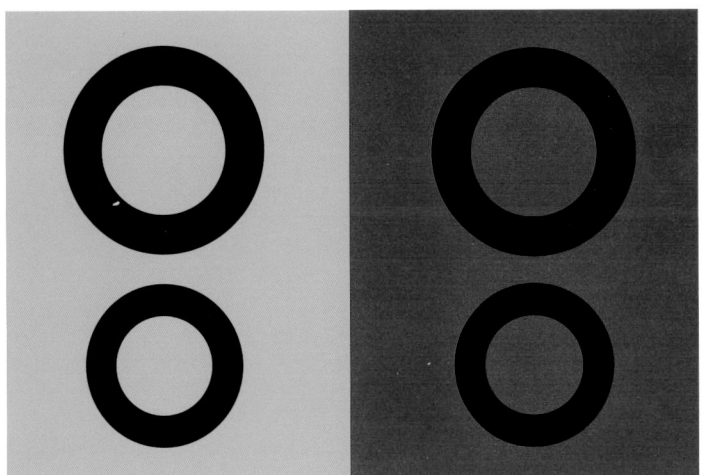

Color Vision

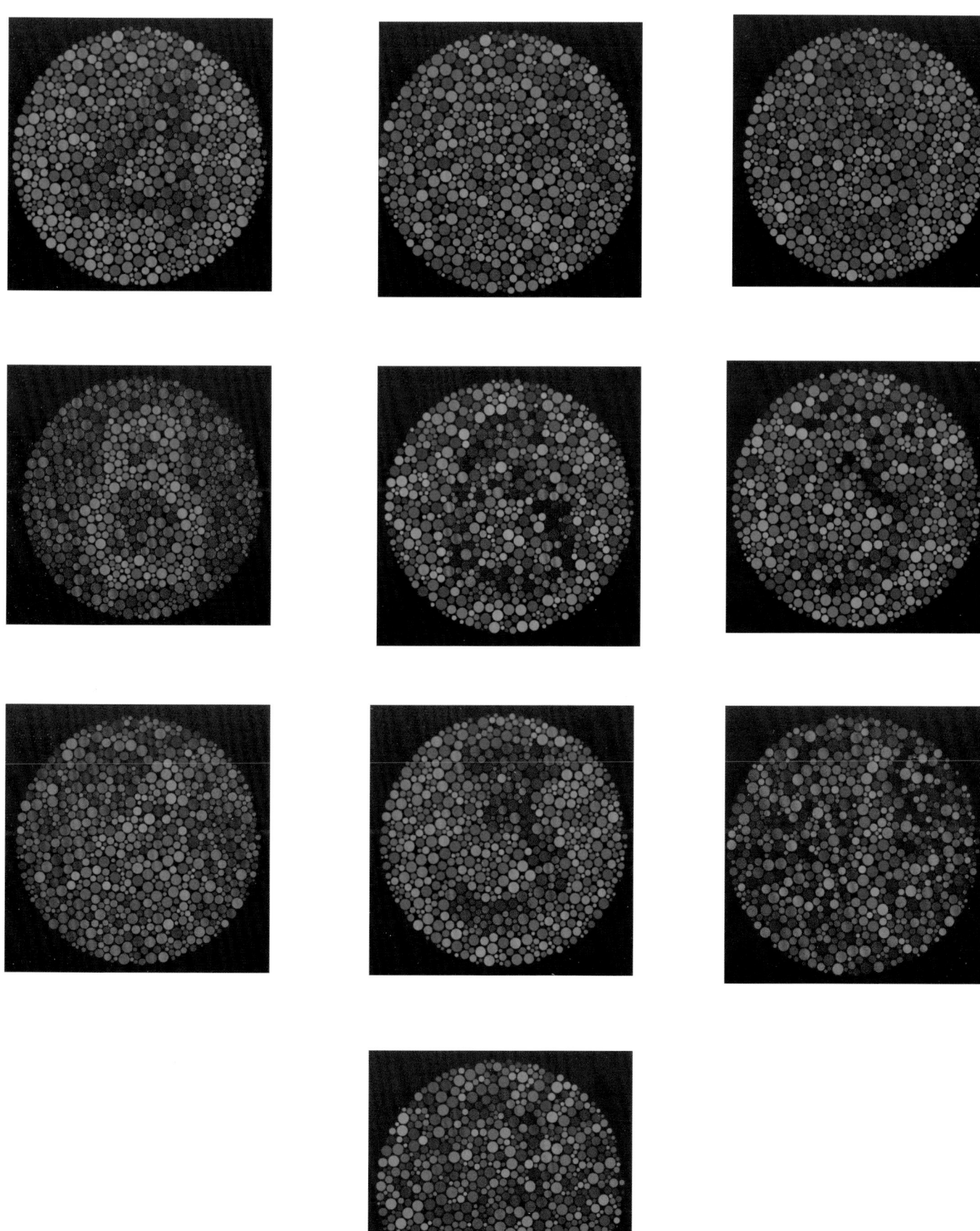

Amsler Grid Test

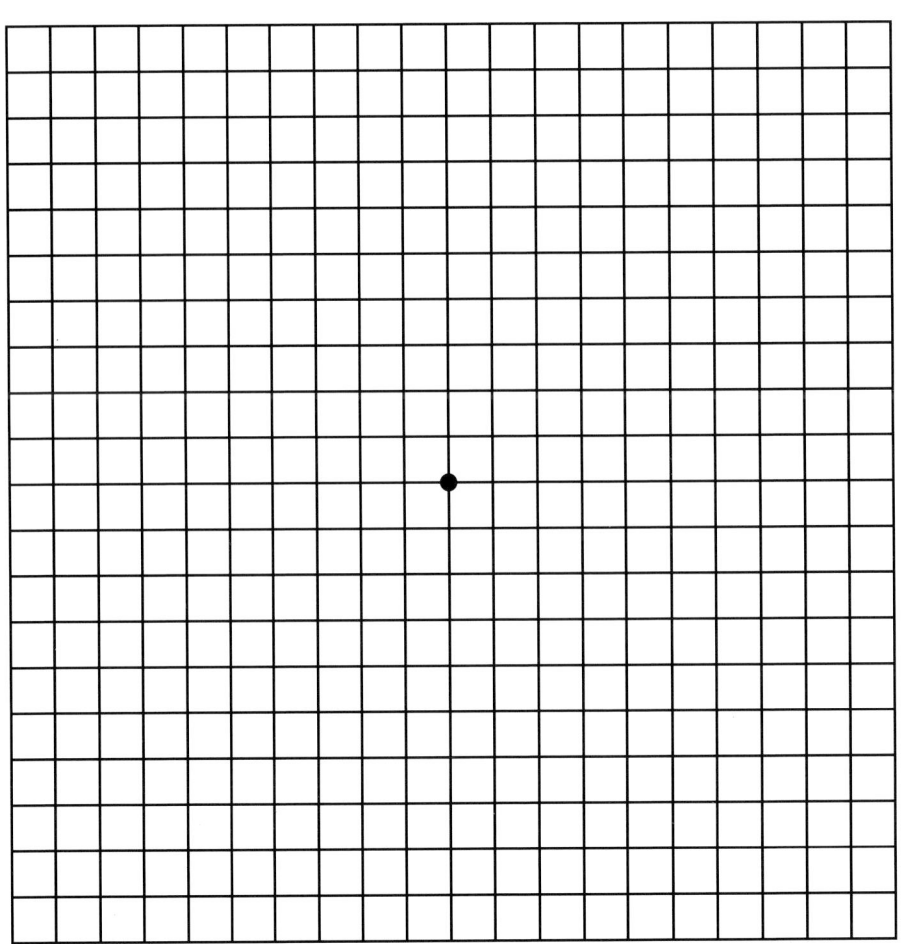

Contrast Vision Test

V R S K D R

N H C S O K

S C N O Z V

C N H Z O K

Reading Strength Test

	FOCUS	DIOPTER	
If this line is difficult to read, use	32	+1.25	W E A K E R
If this line is difficult to read, use	26	+1.50	
If this line is difficult to read, use	22	+1.75	
If this line is difficult to read, use	20	+2.00	
If this line is difficult to read, use	18	+2,25	S T R O N G E R
If this line is difficult to read, use	16	+2.50	
If this line is difficult to read, use	14	+2.75	
If this line is difficult to read, use	12	+3.25	
If this line is difficult to read, use	10	+4.00	

Convergence Test

Sight is mind and eye coordination.	**Sight is mind and eye coordination.**
12	**12**
It is more mental than physical. The eye sees but the mind must interpret and evaluate what is seen.	It is more mental than physical. The eye sees but the mind must interpret and evaluate what is seen.
11	**11**
There are five basic components of mental sight: curiosity, contrast, comparison, memory and judgment.	There are five basic components of mental sight: curiosity, contrast, comparison, memory and judgment.
10	**10**
Curiosity means intelligent visual searching, that is, looking around just as if you saw everything with perfect clarity.	Curiosity means intelligent visual searching, that is, looking around just as if you saw everything with perfect clarity.
9	**9**
Counting objects and colours is the best way to achieve curiosity.	Counting objects and colours is the best way to achieve curiosity.
8	**8**
Contrast is the gradations of difference between foreground and background.	Contrast is the gradations of difference between foreground and background.
7	**7**
For instance, the print on this chart will appear blacker if you close your eyes for a moment and imagine clearly a sheet of clean, white paper before opening then again.	For instance, the print on this chart will appear blacker if you close your eyes for a moment and imagine clearly a sheet of clean, white paper before opening then again.
6	6
6 Comparison is the evaluation of similarity and difference. A capital "H" and a capital "N" both have two parallel sides; but the "H" has a horizontal bar, while the "N" has a diagonal line.	6 Comparison is the evaluation of similarity and difference. A capital "H" and a capital "N" both have two parallel sides; but the "H" has a horizontal bar, while the "N" has a diagonal line.
5	5
Memory is the sum total of our learned and our recollected experiences.	Memory is the sum total of our learned and our recollected experiences.
4	4
Judgment is the summation, the end result, the interpretation or evaluation of what the eye sees.	Judgment is the summation, the end result, the interpretation or evaluation of what the eye sees.
3	3
Always use daylight whenever possible. When reading or working at night be sure to have adequate light consisting of the full spectrum of colours. The best combination of working light is a halogen pin light w h a dimmer switch illuminating your working area. On the left side an incandescent light and possibly fluorescent light fixtures in the ceiling. Fluorescent light alone is the worst working light as far as your eyesight is concerned.	Always use daylight whenever possible. When reading or working at night be sure to have adequate light consisting of the full spectrum of colours. The best combination of working light is a halogen pin light w h a dimmer switch illuminating your working area. On the left side an incandescent light and possibly fluorescent light fixtures in the ceiling. Fluorescent light alone is the worst working light as far as your eyesight is concerned.

Fusion Test

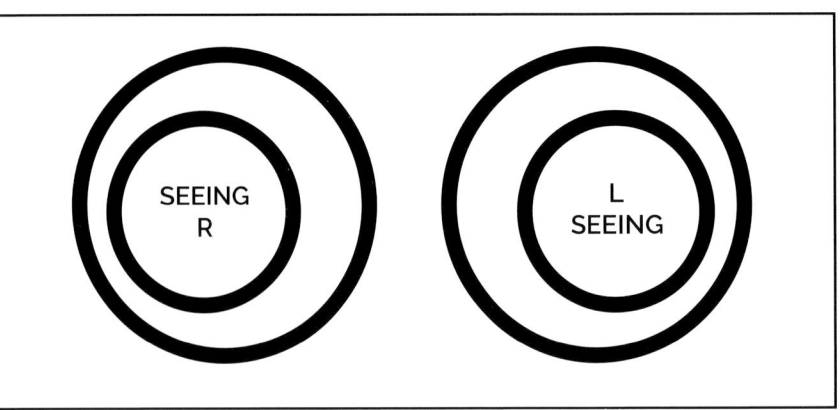

This is what you should see:

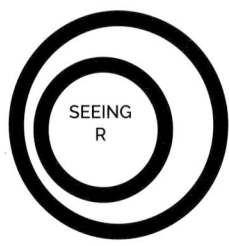 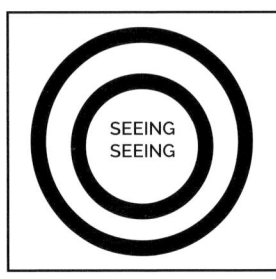 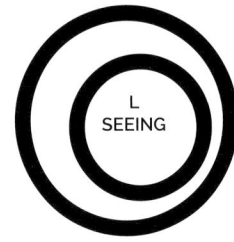

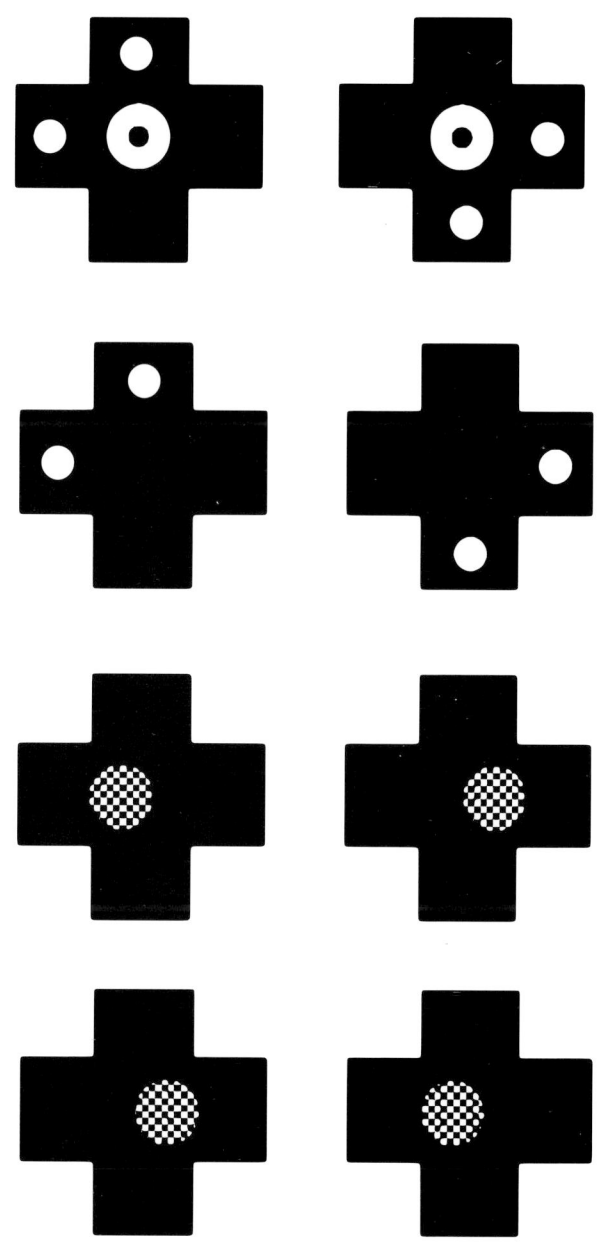